Intercultural Arts Therapies Research

Intercultural Arts Therapies Research: Issues and methodologies is the first overarching study on intercultural practice and research models in the arts therapies. It provides a new departure from traditional arts therapies education and research in that it focuses on research studies only. Written by international experts in the field, the book offers a selection of diverse research undertaken within four arts therapies modalities: art, dance, drama and music.

Drawing on methodologies such as ethnography, phenomenology and case-study research, chapters focus on cultural identity, the transposition of cultural practices to a different context, and the implications of different languages for arts therapies and disability culture. With reference to primary research, it aims to help practitioners and students to develop further research, by making the mechanics of the research process explicit and transparent.

Intercultural Arts Therapies Research will appeal to arts therapists, psychological therapy practitioners, postgraduate students and other health and social care professionals. It will also be of interest to students, artists, teachers, social workers and those working for international aid agencies.

Dr Ditty Dokter is the course leader of MA Dramatherapy, Anglia Ruskin University, Cambridge. She has held posts within NHS trusts and universities and is currently affiliated with the KENVAK arts therapies research centre (Netherlands). She also worked in the tertiary sector to support and advocate the integration of clients with learning disabilities and refugees. Her most recent edited publication is (2011) Dramatherapy and Destructiveness.

Dr Margaret Hills de Zárate originally trained as an Art Therapist (Goldsmith's, University of London), as well as in Counselling, Group Theory and Applications at the Scottish Institute of Human Relations (1990–94). She has been awarded a Master's degree in Education from Edinburgh University (1994) and a PhD from Queen Margaret's University (2006). She has also worked extensively in social and mental health services in the UK, Latin America and Eastern Europe.

International Research in the Arts Therapies
A Routledge Book Series
Series Editors: Diane Waller and Sarah Scoble

This series consists of high-level monographs identifying areas of importance across all arts therapy modalities and highlighting international developments and concerns. It presents recent research from countries across the world and contributes to the evidence-base of the arts therapies. Papers which discuss and analyse current innovations and approaches in the arts therapies and arts therapy education are also included.

This series is accessible to practitioners of the arts therapies and to colleagues in a broad range of related professions, including those in countries where arts therapies are still emerging. The monographs should also provide a valuable source of reference to government departments and health services.

Forthcoming Titles

1. *Intercultural Arts Therapies Research*
   Edited by Ditty Dokter and Margaret Hills de Zárate

Intercultural Arts Therapies Research

Issues and methodologies

Edited by
Ditty Dokter and
Margaret Hills de Zárate

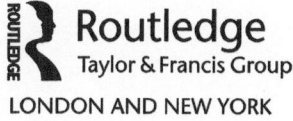
Routledge
Taylor & Francis Group

LONDON AND NEW YORK

British Library Cataloguing in Publication Data
A catalogue record for this book is available from the British Library

Library of Congress Cataloguing in Publication Data
Names: Dokter, Ditty, editor. | Hills De Zárate, Margaret, 1958-
Title: Intercultural arts therapies research: issues and methodologies/edited by Ditty Dokter and Margaret Hills De Zárate.
Description: Abingdon, Oxon; New York, NY: Routledge, 2016.
Identifiers: LCCN 2015046992| ISBN 9781138847842 (hardcover) | ISBN 9781315726441 (electronic)
Subjects: LCSH: Arts – Therapeutic use. | Dance therapy. | Drama – Therapeutic use. | Music therapy.
Classification: LCC RM931.A77 I58 2016 | DDC 616.89/1656 – dc23
LC record available at http://lccn.loc.gov/2015046992

ISBN: 978-1-138-84784-2 (hbk)
ISBN: 978-0-8153-6068-1 (pbk)

Typeset in Bembo
by Florence Production Ltd, Stoodleigh, Devon, UK

Contents

Acknowledgements

The editors Margaret Hills de Zárate and Ditty Dokter would like to acknowledge the assistance of Alexander Hills and David Tatem in the production of
this manuscript.

We thank Sarah Scoble and Diane Waller for asking us to edit this first Ecarte
research series volume, and Heidi Lee, our Routledge editor for her help.

Alexia Quin and Cathy Rowland wish to acknowledge the impact of a
number of skill-sharing projects, which have been implemented by volunteer
music therapists working with *Music as Therapy International*. These therapists
have also played a critical role in the strategic decisions of the charity, as
members of the charity's Advisory Panel, and in devising and developing a range
of training materials and tools. We are indebted to their commitment and hard
work. We would like to specifically thank Caroline Anderson, Liz Coombes,
Nicky Haire, Hannah Hulin and Becca Sayers for undertaking the field work
we refer to in this chapter and Professor Susan Rowland for her guidance in
writing it up.

In volumes such as this, research participants and clients merit thanks in all
their anonymity; without their cooperation research and thus publications such
as this would not be possible.

Ditty Dokter and Margaret Hills de Zárate
August 2015

Chapter 1

Introduction

Ditty Dokter and Margaret Hills de Zárate

Context

The European Consortium for Arts Therapies Education (ECArTE 2015; Kossolapow *et al.* 2001) has been developing arts-therapy education and research since 1991. This volume provides a new departure, in that it focuses on research studies only. The volume consists of nine papers, representing the diversity of research undertaken within four arts-therapy modalities (art, dance, drama and music). They focus on cultural identity: the transposition of cultural practices to a different context, and the implications of different languages for arts therapies and disability culture. The studies draw on such research methodologies as ethnography, phenomenology and case-study research.

The aim is to present a range of a research methodologies and research questions as an initial overview of the types of research in process or completed. They are based around European perspectives, even though – given the diversity represented within the broad term 'European' – this will expand beyond its borders, such as the research into Italian transgenerational migration in South America by Hills de Zárate; or studying the interaction between majority visual and minority tactual culture by Herrmann. These two art-therapy papers are contrasted with the dramatherapy perspectives on drama-therapist cultural identity provided through language (Carr), general therapist cultural background in interaction with that of the client's (Dokter) and teacher/supervisor interaction with an Irish migrant identity (Mullen-Williams). The music therapy perspectives look at importing an 'Eastern' instrumentarium into a 'Western' context (Loth), while conversely exporting the Western model of music therapy outside its borders (Quin and Rowland). The latter's emphasis on training is echoed in the study of trainee diversity in dance therapy (Panhofer *et al.*) and the involvement of a dance therapist in the development of a creative play intervention in isolated Serbia during and post the former-Yugoslavian war in the 1990s. In choosing these papers we aim to present the breadth of intercultural arts-therapy research undertaken, in the hope that further volumes will expand on this beyond European borders as well as within them. In the current (2015) 'migrant/refugee crisis' in Europe, intercultural understanding and interventions are part of a growing need for intercultural connection and communication. Some chapters were selected to study diversity within states, sub-cultures within cultures, others to look at the international phenomenon of student migration, as distinct from war- and poverty-driven migration.

This is the first overarching book on arts-therapy intercultural practice research. Since their inception, arts-therapy pioneers have incorporated intercultural contexts in relation to practice and training in the therapies (Waller 1998, 2009; Jennings 1995, 1997). Arts-therapy volumes have highlighted intercultural practice through case studies, in edited volumes such as *Tapestry of Cultural Issues in Art Therapy* (Hiscox and Calisch 1998), *Arts Therapists, Refugees and Migrants* (Dokter 1998) and *Art Therapy, Race and Culture* (Campbell *et al.* 1999). More recent volumes incorporate both research and practice (Howie *et al.* 2013; Myers & Brooke 2015). Hogan's work, both research- and practice-based (2015, 2012), is broadly in the area of arts-therapy and cultural studies. Bobby Lloyd and Debra Kalmanovitz (2005) wrote about their practice with refugees and war-displaced people, and also about practice development in particular continents, such as Asia (Kalmanovitz 2012). Several useful art-therapy research articles were published by Hocoy (2006, 2005, 2002). In South America several volumes have been published about drama- and arts-therapy practice but do not address research; some are only available in Spanish (Marxen 2011; Martinez 2009; Klein 2006; Fernandez Cao 2006), others in English (Figusch 2006). Several chapters are published in general-practice volumes (e.g. Dokter and Khasnavis 2008; Carr & Andersen 2012; Chang 2009; Hogan 2015), some journal articles (e.g. Hervey and Stuart 2012; Mereni 1996, 1997; Hocoy 2006) or special editions devoted to intercultural issues (*The Arts in Psychotherapy* 1997; *Dramatherapy* 2010). Other important texts, which address intercultural work undertaken with refugee populations in situations of political conflict, are those by Lloyd and Kalmanovitz (1997) and Lloyd and Kalmanowitz, D (eds.) (2005). There are unfortunately too many to mention all of them here, though few are research-based. Those that are relevant are identified in relation to the individual modalities in the chapters.

This introductory chapter defines the arts therapies as used by the chapter authors. We aim to place them in the context of some of those currently used by professional associations. We then define how we use the concepts of culture – intercultural, multicultural, cross-cultural – and how we understand the cultural contexts of arts-therapy practice.

We conclude this introduction by outlining the content of the chapters in this volume. The focus is on the research methodologies used to study intercultural arts-therapy practice.

The arts therapies: definitions

Jones (2005) highlights the need for different definitions to meet different demands: 'There is no single overarching definition that is widely used, but instead there is a lively, rigorous diversity meeting different situations and needs' (Jones 2005: 15). Some definitions are needed for national and global contexts to establish services or define a broad spectrum covering music, drama, dance and art. The more focused definitions tend to relate to working with specific client groups. This approach is particularly useful in an intercultural context, as it both paints a broad picture and shows how different arts therapists and their clients understand their practice in different countries.

The National Coalition of Creative Arts Therapies Associations, founded in 1979, is an alliance of professional associations dedicated to the advancement of the arts as therapeutic modalities.

> Creative arts therapists are human service professionals who use arts modalities and creative processes for the purpose of ameliorating disability and illness and optimizing health and wellness. Treatment outcomes include, for example, improving communication and expression, and increasing physical, emotional, cognitive and/or social functioning.
>
> (NCCATA 2015)

The NCCATA notes commonalities and differences in its focus on the individual arts modalities, while an organization like the International Expressive Arts Therapy Association (IEATA 2015) brings the arts together under one denominator, namely 'expressive'. In the Netherlands the individual arts therapies have united under one professional association (FVB 2015), while in the UK different individual associations have become established in working together on common areas via their registration under the Health and Care Professions Council (HCPC 2015).

The authors in this volume use the following definitions for their individual practice.

The music therapy definition used by Quin and Rowland in Chapter 8 is from Bruscia almost 20 years ago. Music therapy is seen as a systematic process of intervention whereby the therapist helps the client achieve health using musical experiences, and the relationships that develop through them, as dynamic forces of change (Bruscia 1998). Loth in Chapter 5 emphasizes the UK context when she highlights that music therapy practice in the UK is grounded in improvisation and live music-making, while also making use of pre-composed and recorded music (British Association for Music Therapy 2012).

Williams in Chapter 5 refers to the British Association of Dramatherapists definition (BADth 2015), but summarizes her perspective on dramatherapy as one of the HCPC-registered arts therapies that utilizes the medium of the arts to explore a client's material. It is the application of art forms within a relationship between therapist and client for therapeutic benefit. This is a more British emphasis (BADth 2015); the North American Dramatherapy American Association definition (NADTA 2015) stresses the dramatic means more when dramatherapy is defined as an active, experiential approach to facilitating change. Through storytelling, projective play, purposeful improvisation and performance, participants are invited to rehearse desired behaviours, practise being in a relationship, expand and find flexibility between life roles, and perform the change they wish to achieve and see in the world. The emphasis on the (psycho)therapeutic relationship is also echoed in art therapy and dance movement therapy.

The British Association of Art Therapy website (BAAT 2015) defines art therapy as a form of psychotherapy, which uses art media as its primary mode of expression and communication. Within this context, art is not used as diagnostic tool but as a medium to address emotional issues that may be confusing and distressing. The American Art Therapy Association (www.arttherapy.org) defines art therapy as a mental health profession in which clients, facilitated by the art therapist, use art media, the creative process and the resulting artwork to explore their feelings, reconcile emotional conflicts, foster self-awareness, manage behaviour and addictions, develop social skills, improve reality orientation, reduce anxiety and increase self-esteem. A goal in art therapy is to improve or restore a client's functioning and sense of personal wellbeing.

The Association for Dance Movement Psychotherapy in the UK (ADMPUK) emphasizes body movement as an implicit and expressive instrument of communication and expression. Dance movement psychotherapy (ADMPUK 2015) is a relational process in which client/s and therapist engage creatively using body movement and dance to assist integration of emotional, cognitive, physical, social and spiritual aspects of self. The philosophical orientation of Dance Movement Psychotherapy (DMP) is based on the intrinsic belief in the inter-relationship between psyche, soma and spirit, as evidenced in the potential held in creative processes. The European Association (EADMT 2015) stresses that the intervention aims to offer individuals of *all* ages and abilities a space to explore what drives them, assisting people to develop self-awareness and sensitivity to others and also to find a pathway to feeling more comfortable in their own skin.

Definitions of arts therapy can emphasize the arts form or relationship, be it generalizing or focusing. However, there is a need to understand the dominant Western values that have influenced arts-therapy practice (Kalmanovitz *et al.* 2012; Hocoy 2002, 2005, 2006; Hogan 2015; Hogan & Pink 2010). This volume aims to situate research related to identity and difference within larger historical and social contexts (Talwar 2010) and to evaluate the strengths and weaknesses of research methodologies used to study these issues.

Concepts of culture, intercultural, cross-cultural, multicultural, trans-cultural

Definitions of culture bring a similar need to explore diversity as in defining the arts therapies. Halford (2006: 9) notes 'the concept of culture is so indeterminate that it can be easily filled in with whatever preconceptions a theorist brings to it'. Krause (1998: 174) acknowledges that culture is dynamic, 'always changing and shifting and in the process of being created'. People can be seen as belonging to several, or indeed many, cultures (Gil & Drewes 2005). From a therapeutic point of view, Blackwell sees culture as 'the symbolic universe of its members' (2005: 38) and 'the organization of collective human life and, indeed, of the meaning of life. And these meanings are internalized in the individual ego or self.' People are not necessarily aware of their own cultural values and assumptions: 'we see the world and each other through our own cultural filters' (Dokter 1998: 147).

In defining culture, Stuart Hall follows Raymond Williams by describing it as 'those patterns of organization, those characteristic forms of human energy which can be discovered as revealing themselves . . . within or underlying *all* social practices' (Hall 1986: 36).

Interculturality derives from the understanding that cultures thrive only in contact with other cultures, not in isolation (COE 2014). Intercultural psychotherapy is a term used in the UK context (Kareem & Littlewood 1992) to indicate the interactive element in cultural dynamics between the different parties involved in therapy. Cultural differences refer to variations in attitudes, values and perceptual constructs that result from different cultural experiences (Zane *et al.* 2004).

The Council of Europe (COE) contrasts interculturalism with assimilationist approaches, which seek to obscure and ultimately eradicate diversity. This is supported by Samovar, Porter and McDaniel (2011) who point out the limits to cultural diversity and the importance of belonging. Similarly, Scollon, Scollon and Jones (2011) propose to replace the concept 'culture' with the concept 'discourse systems', in order to eliminate problematic overgeneralizations and oversimplifications. Scollon *et al.* (2000) also replace 'intercultural communication' with 'interdiscursive communication' since, according to these authors, cultures do not interact, but individuals and discourses do.

In addition, the COE contrasts interculturalism with multiculturalism, which has, according to COE, overemphasized diversity. Similarly, Vertovec and Wessendorf (2010) provide a critique of multiculturalism when emphasized as a singular, fixed ideology or dogma, announcing its slow death. Many immigrants, encouraged by multicultural orthodoxy, retreat into their differentness, they claim. Thus, multiculturalism fosters separateness and denies common values.

By taking the object as its focus, the relationship between memory and the material world is explored in relation to cultural translation conceived as relating to processes that are not exclusively inter-lingual (between languages) but also those processes that are intermedial (between media) or intercultural (between cultures) and encompass issues such as the 'untranslatable', and the impact of what is transformed, gained or lost in the process of translation (Forsdick 2014).

Transnationalism is the idea that flows of trans-state migrants and their symbolic and material accoutrements are bi- or multi-directional and ongoing. That is, where previous generations of migrants tended towards making a 'clean break' with their societies of origin, many contemporary migrants continue to have ongoing ties with the communities from which they migrated. Transnationalism has been defined in anthropology as 'the process by which immigrants forge and sustain simultaneous multi-stranded social relations that link together their societies of origin and settlement. . . . Many immigrants today build social fields that cross geo-graphic, cultural and political borders' (King 2005: 2220–2221).

Although both terms refer to cross-border processes, diaspora has been often used to denote religious or national groups living outside an (imagined) homeland, whereas transnationalism is often used both more narrowly – to refer to migrants' durable ties across countries – and more widely, to capture not only communities but all sorts of social formations, such as transnationally active networks, groups and organizations. Moreover, while diaspora and trans-nationalism are sometimes used interchangeably, the two terms reflect different intellectual genealogies (Bauböck *et al.* 2005).

Intercultural arts-therapy research has been strongly influenced by both cultural studies (Hall 1986) and cultural anthropology. In a retrospective view of cultural anthropology, for example, Clifford Geertz (2002) said that from the mid-1960s through to the end of the 1970s, different paradigms of analysis flowered, including French structuralism, sociobiology, cognitive anthropology, the ethnography of speaking, cultural materialism, neo-Marxism, neo-evolutionism, functionalism, practice theory, the anthropology of experience, subaltern studies and interpretive anthropology. He adds feminism, anti-imperialism, indigenous rights and gay liberation (Rosaldo 2005).

Overview of content

The book is divided into three parts: intercultural communication, good practice guidelines and skills sharing, and, finally, ethnographic voices.

The first four chapters concern the use of language in dramatherapy, especially when the therapist, client or both work in a second language. Through phenomenological interviewing methodology a number of themes emerge, including the implications of verbal language being understood, whether the arts function as languages in themselves, the challenges of working with interpreters, issues of language, power and culture, the dynamic between language and the therapeutic process and, finally, the use of mother tongue within dramatherapy. It is suggested that opportunities and challenges may include whether to offer clients the chance to work in their mother tongue, how to work with interpreters, a consideration of potential links between psychoanalytical concepts and language issues, as well as the power dynamic between therapist and client and its implications for the negotiation of meaning within dramatherapy.

Uwe Herrmann's chapter shows how, when the blind client and the sighted art therapist engage in therapy, their respective visual and tactile cultures highlight their sensory, psychological and aesthetic differences. While practice engenders these differences, researching the blind–sighted encounter in arts therapy pinpoints the separate cultures on a methodological, aesthetic and theoretical level. Herrmann presents arts-therapy research as an aesthetic and methodical endeavour that places the art in arts therapy centre stage and explores how collaborative research with blind clients can lead to devising visual and tactile enquiry methods that consider distinct sensory cultures.

Two dance therapists and a group analyst use the ethnographic-inquiry method to study intercultural dynamics in a large experiential group during postgraduate training using phenomenographic-research methodology. This methodological framework stems from a basic original objective, which is to describe a single session of an experiential group from the point of view of all of its participants. The research goal is to generate a multi-subjective description of a single learning experience. The findings show that a diverse group, working within a complex academic context, tends to evolve a micro-culture, manifest within the large group, in which cultural differences are not expressed and are perhaps avoided by the students. Instead, groups and sub-groups are formed around different criteria within the university setting.

The final chapter in the intercultural communication section focuses on the use of the gamelan in music therapy. The use of music and instruments from different cultures in music therapy practice is an area that has not been widely investigated. Some music therapists have considered the relevance of importing Western music therapy and its inherent music and instruments to non-Western cultures; however, there is little research into bringing non-Western music to Western music therapy practice. This chapter describes research into how the music and instruments from one culture can be taken and used for therapeutic purposes in a different one. It is based on a research study into the relevance of Indonesian gamelan music to music therapy practice in the UK. The chapter shows how the cultural aspects of gamelan music can be transposed into Western music therapy practice. The possibilities, as well as the difficulties, arising from this transposition are discussed.

The second part of the book looks at the development of intercultural good practice guidelines in dramatherapy, using such research methodologies as survey and audit, as well as vignette and other collaborative methods. The chapter highlights aspects of therapist and client background affecting the therapeutic relationship. Quin and Rowland's chapter outlines and explores some of the different skill-sharing models used by the British charity Music as Therapy International in a number of different countries. The charity's roots lie in the institutions in Romania, where it developed a six-week model within which UK music therapists worked alongside local practitioners. The chapter evaluates the impact of the training programme and describes a portfolio of training activities that have been developed and adapted to embrace local cultural norms. The challenges and impact of this approach to skill sharing are discussed.

Three different ethnographic chapters complete the volume. Singer has researched the impact of post-war work in Serbia and analyses the different voices of the Serbian psychologist co-researchers in dialogue with the UK Dance Ethnographer/dance and dramatherapist. Italian intergenerational migration in South America and the role of material culture is researched by Margaret Hills de Zárate, while Julianne Mullen uses auto-ethnography to analyse the impact of her Irish migrant background on her research into dramatherapy supervision methods impacting on newly qualified teachers in the UK.

These final authors make use of ethnographic methodologies, a cultural practice, as is the practice of the arts therapies where the reflective and reflexive processes in which we engage allow us to be self-critical and ethical in our clinical practice, nurturing our development as therapists and sustaining our practice-based learning (Stedmon & Dallos 2009).

As editors we are aiming for this book to encourage this reflective process. We are hoping that the development of intercultural good practice guidelines will lead to further research, so that guidelines can become more evidence-based, whether practice-based evidence or evidence-based practice. If arts-therapy research in general were to incorporate cultural-background monitoring as a routine aspect of research projects, currently invisible data could be made visible. The research methodology in this volume is mostly qualitative, reflecting a broader tendency in arts-therapy research. If we are to address the full range of questions relating to intercultural practice, we will need to use the full range of methodologies available. Worldwide exchange and engagement between arts-therapy researchers, and collaboration with researchers from other disciplines such as nursing, medicine, cultural studies, linguistics and education are happening in all of the arts-therapy modalities, and this can be built upon to achieve a much broader and better evidence base for intercultural arts-therapy research.

Bibliography

ADMT – Association for Dance Movement Psychotherapy UK. Available online at: www.admt.org.uk (accessed 27 July 2015).

ARTTHERAPY – American Art Therapy Association. Available online at: www. arttherapy.org (accessed 27 July 2015).

BAAT – British Association of Art Therapists. Available online at: www.baat.org (accessed 27 July 2015).

BADth – British Association of Dramatherapists. Available online at: www.badth.org.uk (accessed 27 July 2015).

BAMT – British Association for Music Therapy. Available online at: www.bamt.org (accessed 27 July 2015).

Bauböck, R. & Faist, T. (2005), *Diaspora and Transnationalism: concepts, theories and methods*, Amersterdam, The Netherlands: IMISCOE-Amsterdam University.

Blackwell, D. (2005), *Counselling and Psychotherapy with Refugees*, London and Philadelphia: Jessica Kingsley.

Bruscia, K. (1998), *Defining Music Therapy*, (2nd edn.), Barcelona: Gilsum NH.

Campbell, J., Liebmann, M., Brooks, F. Jones, J. & Ward, C. (eds.) (1999), *Art Therapy, Race and Culture*, London: Jessica Kingsley.

Carr, M. (2012), 'Romeo and Juliet and Dramatic Distancing: chaos and anger contained for inner city adolescents in multicultural schools', in Leigh, L., Gersch, I., Dix, A., Haythorne, D. (eds.) *Dramatherapy with Children, Young People and Schools: enabling creativity, sociability, communication and learning* (pp. 91–7), London: Routledge.

Carr, M. & Andersen-Warren, M. (2012), 'Clinical Comment – A Research Interview: dramatherapy and cross-cultural awareness', *Journal of the British Association of Dramatherapists*, 34 (2): 92–100.

Chang, M. (2009), 'Cultural Consciousness and the Global Context of Dance Movement Therapy', in Chaiklin, S. & Wengrower, H. (eds.) *The Art and Science of Dance Movement Therapy*, New York and Hove, East Sussex: Taylor & Francis.

COE – Intercultural City: Governance and policies for diverse communities, The Council of Europe. Available online at: www.coe.int/t/dg4/cultureheritage/culture/Cities/Interculturality_en.pdf (accessed 28 October 2014).

Dokter, D. (1998), *Arts Therapists, Refugees and Migrants: reaching across borders*, London: Jessica Kingsley.

Dokter, D. & Khasnavis, R. (2008), 'Intercultural Supervision: the issue of choice', in P. Jones & D. Dokter (eds.) *Supervision of Dramatherapy* (pp. 111–129), London: Routledge.

EADMT– The European Association Dance Movement Therapy. Available online at: www.eadmt.com (accessed 27 July 2015).

ECArTE – European Consortium of Arts Therapies Educators. Available online at: www.ecarte.info (accessed 27 July 2015).

FVB – Federatie Vaktherapeutische Beroepen (FVB). Available online at: www.vaktherapie.nl (accessed 27 July 2015).

Geertz, G. (2002), 'An inconstant profession: the anthropological life in interesting times', *Annual Review of Anthropology*, 31: 1–19.

Gil, E. & Drewes, A. (eds.) (2005), *Cultural Issues in Play Therapy*, London and New York: Guilford.

Hall, S. (1986), 'Cultural Studies: two paradigms', in R. Collins, J. Curran, N. Garnham, N. Scannell, P. Schlesinger & C. Sparks (eds.) *Media, Culture and Society: A Critical Reader* (pp.35–6), London: Sage.

Health and Care Professions Council. Available online at: www.hcpc.org.uk (accessed 27 July 2015).

Hervey, L. & Stuart, L. (2012), 'Multi cultural competency education in the ADTA approved graduate programs', *American Journal of Dance Therapy*, 34: 85–98.

Hills de Zárate, M. (2010), Tropical Path (Part 1) (English version) *ATOL: Art Therapy Online*, 1 (1). Available online at: http://journals.gold.ac.uk/119/3/Hill_Tropical.pdf (accessed 27 August 2015).

Hills de Zárate, M. (2011), Tropical Path (Part 2), *ATOL: Art Therapy Online*, 1 (2). Available online at: http://journals.gold.ac.uk/249/1/Tropical_Path_Part_2.pdf (accessed 27 August 2015).

Hiscox, A.R. & Calisch, A.C. (eds.) (1998), *Tapestry of Cultural Issues in Art Therapy*, London: Jessica Kingsley.

Hocoy, D. (2002), 'Cross-cultural Issues in Art Therapy', *Art Therapy: Journal of the American Art Therapy Association*, 19 (4): 141–5.

Hocoy, D. (2005), 'Ethnography as metaphor in psychotherapy training', *American Journal of Psychotherapy*, 59 (2): 101–18.

Hocoy, D. (2006) 'Art Therapy: working in the borderlands', *Art Therapy: Journal of the American Art Therapy Association*, 23 (3): 132–5.

Hogan, S. (2015a), 'Lost in Translation? Inter-Cultural Exchange', in C.E. Myers & Brooke, S.L. (eds.) *Therapists Creating a Cultural Tapestry Using the Creative Therapies Across Cultures* (pp. 11–25), Springfield, Il: Charles C. Thomas.

Hogan, S. (2015b), 'Interrogating Women's Experience of Ageing – Reinforcing or Challenging Clichés?', *The International Journal of the Arts in Society: Annual Review*, 9: 1–18.

Hogan, S. & Pink, S. (2010), 'Routes to Interiorities: art therapy and knowing in anthropology', *Visual Anthropology*, 23: 158–74.

Hogan, S. & Warren, L. (2013), 'Women's Inequality: A Global Problem Explored in Participatory Arts. International Perspectives on Research-Guided Practice in Community-Based Arts in Health', Special Issue *UNESCO Observatory*, 3 (3): 1–27.

Howie, P., Prasad, S. & Kristel, J. (eds.) (2013), *Using Art Therapy with Diverse Populations Crossing Cultures and Abilities*. London: Jessica Kingsley.

International Expressive Arts Therapy Association (IEATA). Available online at: www.ieata.org (accessed 27 June 2015).

Jennings, S. (1995), *Theatre, Ritual and Transformation: The Senoi Temiar*, London: Routledge.

Jennings, S. (1997) *Dramatherapy Theory and Practice 3*, London: Routledge.

Jones, P. (2005), *The Arts Therapies: a revolution in health care*, London: Routledge.

Kalmanovitz, D., Jordan, S. & Siu mei C. (eds.) (2012), *Art Therapy in Asia: To the bone or wrapped in silk*, London: Jessica Kingsley.

Kareem J. & Littlewood. R. (1992), *Intercultural Therapy*, Oxford: Blackwell.

King, D.E. (2005), *Encyclopedia of Anthropology*, London: Sage.

Kossolapow, L., Scoble, S. & Waller, D. (eds.) (2001), *Arts – Therapies – Communication?: on the way to a communicative European arts therapy*, Münster: LIT Verlag.

Krause, I. (1998), *Therapy Across Culture*, London: Sage.

Lloyd, B. & Kalmanovitz, D. (1997), *The Portable Studio?: art therapy and political conflict, initiatives in former Yugoslavia and KwaZulu-Natal, South Africa?*, London: Health Education England.

Lloyd, B. & Kalmanovitz, D. (2005), *Art Therapy and Political Violence: with or without illusion*. London: Routledge.

López Fernadez Cao, M. (2011), *Memoria, ausencia e identidad. El arte como Terapia*, Madrid: Eneida.

Martinez Diez, N. (2012), 'Frente a la maldición de Babel. Terapia, arte y migraciones. Arteprosocial en sociedades dinámicas', *Arteterapia: Papeles de arteterapia y educación artística para la inclusión social*, 313 (7): 313–4.

Marxen, E (2004), 'Arteterapia e inmigración', *RTS: Revista de treball social*, ISSN 0212–7210, N°. 173, 2004 (Ejemplar dedicado a: La inmigración, nuevos vecinos, nuevas oportunidades): 71–6.

Marxen, E. (2008), 'Kunsttherapie und Immigration', in R. Hampe & P.B. Stalder (Eds.). *Grenzüberschreitungen. Bewusstseinswandel und Gesundheitshandeln* (pp. 269–73). Berlin: Frank & Timme.

Marxen, E. (2009), 'La etnografía desde el arte Definiciones, bases teóricas y nuevos escenarios', *Alteridades*, 19 (37): 7–22.

Marxen, E. (2010), 'Le symbolisme culturel spécifique et le rythme: thérapie d'une femme marocaine', *La Revue Francaise de Musicotherapie*, XXX (4): 43–52.

Marxen, E (2011), *Diálogos entre arte y terapia: Del 'arte psicótico' al desarrollo de la arteterapia y sus aplicaciones*, Barcelona: Gedisa.

Mereni, A.E. (1996), 'Kinesis and katharsis I', *British Journal of Music Therapy* 10 (1) 17–23.

Mereni, A.E. (1997), 'Kinesis and katharsis II, *British Journal of Music Therapy* 11 (1) 20–3.

Myers, C.E. & Brooke, S.L. (eds.) (2015), *Therapists creating a cultural tapestry using the creative therapiues across cultures*, Springfield, IL: Charles C. Thomas.

National Coalition for Creative Arts Therapies Associations – NCCATA. Available online at: www.ncacta.org (accessed 27 July 2015).

North American Drama Therapy Association (NADTA). Available online at: www.nadta.org (accessed 27 July 2015).

Rico Caballo, L. (2012), *Frente a la maldición de Babel. Terapia, arte y mi- graciones. Arteprosocial en sociedades dinámicas*, Madrid: Editorial Psimatica.

Rosaldo, R. (2005), 'Foreword', in Baldwin, J.R.,Faulkner, S.L., Hecht, M.L., Lindsley, S.L. (eds.) *Redefining Culture: Perspectives across the disciplines* (pp. ix–xiv), London: Routledge.

Samovar, L., Porter, R. & McDaniel, E. (2011), *Intercultural Communication: A reader*, Wadsworth, MA: Cengage Learning.

Scollon, R. (2000), 'Methodological Interdiscursivity: An Ethnographic Understanding of Unfinalisability', in Sarangi, S. & Coulthard, M. (2000), *Discourse and Social Life* (pp. 138–54), Abingdon and New York: Routledge.

Scollon, R., Scollon, S.W. & Jones, R.H. (2011), *Intercultural Communication: a discourse approach* (3rd edn.), Oxford: Wiley Blackwell.

Stedmon, J. & Dallos, R. (2009), *Reflective Practice in Psychotherapy and Counselling*, Maidenhead and New York: Open University Press: McGraw-Hill Education.

Talwar, S. (2010), 'An intersectional framework for race, class, gender and sexuality in art therapy,' *Art Therapy Journal of the American Art Therapy Association*, 27 (1): 11–17.

Vertovec, S. & Wessendorf, S. (eds.) (2010), *The Multiculturalism Backlash: European discourses, policies and practices*, London: Routledge.

Waller, D. (1998), *Towards a European Art Therapy: Creating a profession*, Open University.

Waller, D. (2009), 'The Influence of Culture on Aesthetic Preferences', in H.O. Thomashoff and E. Sukhanova, E (eds.) *The Person in Art* (pp. 57–69), New York: Nova.

Part I

Communication and culture

Chapter 2

Dramatherapy across languages

Experiences, drawbacks and opportunities for dramatherapists and their clients, working in a second language

Mandy Carr

> *You ask me what I mean*
> *by saying I have lost my tongue.*
> *I ask you, what would you do*
> *if you had two tongues in your mouth,*
> *and lost the first one, the mother tongue, and could not really know the other,*
> *the foreign tongue.*

(Bhatt 2013: 48)

Introduction

Given the increasingly multilingual and multicultural nature of UK society, this chapter aims to explore the dynamics and meaning that may emerge in the dramatherapeutic encounter where bilingualism or multilingualism is significant. Identity is neither static nor immutable, and language is often seen as a crucial element of identity (Skutnabb-Kangas 1981). The lines from Bhatt's poem 'Search for my Tongue', which introduce this chapter, express a sense of profound loss that can be experienced when functioning in a second language on a daily basis. The use of mother tongue can be fraught with emotional complexity (Conci 2010), perhaps associated with the mother's role in trans- mitting a culture, or indeed as the very embodiment of that culture (Mills 2004). The use of the term 'culture' itself can be can be controversial, and is widely acknowledged as difficult to define. Halford, cited in Moodley (2006: 9), notes, 'the concept of culture is so indeterminate that it can be easily filled in with whatever preconceptions a theorist brings to it'. Krause (1998: 174) acknow- ledges that culture is dynamic, 'always changing and shifting and in the process of being created'. People can be seen as belonging to several, or indeed many, cultures (Gil & Drewes 2005). From a therapeutic point of view, Blackwell sees culture as 'the symbolic universe of its members' (2005: 38). He views culture as 'the organization of collective human life and, indeed, of the mean- ing of life. And these meanings are internalized in the individual ego or self' (2005: 38). People are not necessarily aware of their own cultural values and assumptions (Dokter 1998). Dramatherapist Dokter goes on to suggest, 'we see the world and each other through our own cultural filters' (1998: 147).

From a psychotherapeutic perspective, Frie argues for the inherent connection between language and culture in the therapeutic setting:

> We overlook the degree to which we are *all* inescapably embedded in cultures, histories and languages that are not of our own making. Each of us is born into and emerges into a cultural context of language and social practice. Language and speech situate us in family, history and tradition.
>
> (2013: 11)

He goes on to argue that language is central to the therapeutic process because 'it enables us to be heard' (2013: 11). This chapter aims to explore whether language is regarded as central to the therapeutic relationship within dramatherapy, or whether the use of the arts is seen somehow as going beyond language. Integrative arts psychotherapist James quotes a client from Ghana, who sees the arts as offering access to many languages: 'The arts can work cross-culturally because they offer so many languages to be able to understand' (1998: 210). Moreover, Braithwaite contends 'educational and therapeutic usage of dance, theatre and music do speak for themselves, during mental/physical health assessment and treatment across cultures' (1998: 191).

This chapter, therefore, examines the experiences of bilingual or multilingual dramatherapists. Following a brief reflexive exploration of the author's background, the study goes on to explain the methodology, as well as summarizing and analysing the themes emerging from an analysis of five interviews. The thematic analysis draws on an interpretative phenomenological approach (IPA), which aims to explore in detail how participants make sense of their personal and social worlds (Smith *et al.* 1999: 218–40). Interviews with practising dramatherapists utilized open questions with the intention of providing 'an understanding of the common experiences of the participants' (Cresswell 2007: 61). Verbatim quotes from dramatherapists aim to give 'snapshots' of their experience, and it is hoped that readers will gain a sense of the authentic voices of the bilingual or multilingual therapists, while anonymity is retained. Discussion of the literature and the findings are interwoven. Finally, possible implications arising from the themes are suggested, followed by a discussion of challenges and opportunities for dramatherapists and clients working in an additional language, and suggestions for practice, training and research.

Reflexivity

My Liberal Jewish childhood not only immersed me in a culture in which social responsibility and addressing inequalities were key values, but also in a multilingual community that included migrants who had escaped from the tyranny of 1930s Nazism in Europe. Diverse attitudes to language were passionately held, ranging from the desire to suppress linguistic identity under a mask of quintessential Englishness to the vital importance of maintaining heritage languages such as Yiddish. In other words, links between language and existential survival itself were major influences in my own development.

Before training as a dramatherapist, I spent 16 years as a Head of English as an Additional Language (EAL) in inner-city London schools, in which it was common for the student population to comprise speakers of forty or more languages. The cornerstone of thinking in EAL pedagogy, from the 1980s to the early twenty-first century, was that opportunities to develop a child's mother tongue were essential for cognitive, linguistic and emotional development. 'Mother tongue promotion in the school helps develop not only the mother tongue itself but also children's abilities in the majority school language' (Cummins 2001: 18). Further, it was believed that expecting a child to function only in English, rather than drawing on their own language or languages, would be equivalent to asking them to leave a central part of themselves outside the school gates: 'To reject a child's language in the school is to reject the child' (Cummins 2001: 18).

Many dramatherapists work in inner-city multilingual settings, some with migrants including recently arrived refugees or asylum seekers. This study looks at dramatherapists' thoughts about affirming the linguistic identity of their clients and their confidence or otherwise in drawing on mother tongue/multilingual experience. My own bias is to a belief in the central importance of the mother tongue to identity, and of affirming clients' linguistic history and repertoire. My own practice includes ensuring that clients can choose to work in their preferred language. I have therefore aimed to 'bracket' my own views as far as possible during the interviews and process of analysis.

Linguistic backgrounds of British dramatherapists

While multilingualism and bilingualism are discussed in the literature of Psychotherapy and Education, relatively little has been written in English within the field of dramatherapy. The British Association of Dramatherapists (BADth) 2015 survey of UK dramatherapists' backgrounds shows that of respondents (51 per cent of the membership), 21.5 per cent were born in countries outside the United Kingdom, in thirty-three different countries.

While there are currently no available data on the linguistic backgrounds of dramatherapists or their clients, this survey indicates that a significant proportion of BADth members come from bilingual or multilingual backgrounds, with English as an additional language. Notably, a slightly higher proportion of UK psychotherapists are bilingual or multilingual. Dewaele and Costa state: 'The current data do not present a very clear picture but where organizations keep data on therapists' multilingualism, the current situation (2013) for active members registered with the United Kingdom Council for Psychotherapy, for example, shows that 1,298 are able to conduct therapy in more than one language out of a total active membership of 7, 085' (2012: 19).

Key terms

This enquiry examines the experiences of dramatherapists working in an additional language. The term 'bilingual' is defined as 'describing someone possessing two languages' (Li Wei 2000: 7). This term can cover any number of languages, and does not describe levels of fluency. The abbreviation L1 (Language 1) is used interchangeably with the term mother tongue (Ball 2011: 8).

Methodology

The interviewees were bilingual dramatherapists who responded to an advertisement in *The Prompt*, the magazine of the British Association of Dramatherapists. Five dramatherapists were interviewed on Skype. Their level of professional experience ranged from 33 years to newly qualified, and included three experienced dramatherapists who had worked in the field for more than twenty years, one who had been qualified for two-and-a-half years and one newly qualified therapist. There were four women and one man, and all the respondents were bilingual or multilingual.

Four were from European countries and one was from North America. All qualified as dramatherapists in the UK. They practised in four European countries, including the UK. They were assured that they would be unidentifiable, and for this reason their particular countries and languages remain anonymous in the research. While this may diminish the sense of context, it perhaps enabled the respondents to speak more freely about their experiences. The interviewees were offered a draft of the article, to check that they were happy with their anonymity and also that their experiences had been accurately represented in the text.

The interviews were recorded and transcribed. IPA acknowledges that researchers and participants are involved in a dynamic process, informed also by their cultural and social contexts. The interviews were listened to and the transcripts were read several times in the hope of gaining insight into any researcher bias and to ensure as far as possible that description and analysis were firmly based on the data. Themes were selected if three out of five respondents mentioned them. Selected points made by individual interviewees will also be cited, if they seemed to the researcher to have been made emphatically. Data analysis, therefore highlighted 'significant statements, sentences, or quotes that provide an understanding of how the participant experiences the phenomenon' (Cresswell 2007: 61).

As the researcher was aware of her own biases described earlier, particular care was taken in the formulation of questions, the interview and data analysis processes, to ensure, as far as possible, that viewpoints that differed from the author's were fully included. It is hoped that the opportunity for interviewees to check and amend results may further diminish bias.

The research approach is qualitative and no generalizations can be drawn from the findings. Being phenomenological, the aim is to describe the experience of the dramatherapists, 'to search for meanings and essences rather than explanations and utility. It is, therefore, mostly concerned with *description* rather than interpretation' (Zografou 2012: 86). It is hoped that data, along with a discussion of the literature, might stimulate further reflection and new ways of thinking about bilingualism and dramatherapy, as 'the phenomenological literature presented as naïve enquiry is, in fact, the necessary step towards the opening of new possibilities and fresh ideas about life and the human condition' (Zografou 2012: 88).

Data analysis

The data explored the experience of the participants as bilingual dramatherapists, as well as their work with bilingual clients. There were significant differences between the reflections, as well as several emergent themes. The interviews were semi-structured, the questions designed to be as open-ended as possible, in effect 'broadly constructed to allow for unanticipated themes to emerge' (Callary, Rathwell & Young 2015: 63). The respondents were sent the following questions to consider, a few days prior to the interview:

- What is the experience of dramatherapists and clients utilizing a second language?
- What are the implications for the therapeutic relationship?
- Does the use of the arts go beyond language?
- To what extent does the use of interpreters help or hinder the process?
- Do dramatherapists believe it's important to affirm the linguistic identity of their clients?
- How confident are dramatherapists in drawing on the mother tongue/ multilingual experience of the client and does it matter if the therapist does not understand that language?
- Do bilingual/multilingual clients feel more comfortable working with a bilingual/multilingual therapist?

Three main areas of focus emerged: first, their experience as bilingual dramatherapists; second, their own experiences as bilingual clients in therapy; and finally their reflections on their work with bilingual clients.

I Reflections on the experience of bilingual dramatherapists

The dramatherapists were eager to discuss their experiences and covered a wide range of personal and professional experience. Four themes emerged from the data:

Theme 1: The arts as languages themselves vs. the power of spoken language
Theme 2: The importance of being understood/negotiating meaning.
Theme 3: The challenges of working with interpreters.
Theme 4: Power issues/feeling disempowered.

Theme 1: The arts as languages themselves vs. the power of spoken language

All the interviewees spoke powerfully about the arts as languages of their own, but expressed a range of feelings. One practitioner warned of the dangers of devaluing spoken language, while three felt that the arts offer a deeper form of communication than language: 'They go beyond. There is a universal language that is common to all of us.'

A dramatherapist who had worked with a Chinese and an Italian child, both newly arrived in the UK, and at the beginning stages of English learning, reflected: 'When using the arts and play in the sessions, it seemed to tap into another language they already held as part of themselves. It was also their language, they didn't need words. They played all kinds of roles with lots of interaction and eye contact. This may have reduced feelings of isolation as these different languages developed within the group. They could experiment maybe as babies do. The language barrier was maybe suspended or erased in this exploration.'

Three therapists felt emphatically that working through the arts could transcend verbal language, drama being described as a 'bridge between languages' and a 'meeting in the middle using a shared language'. One respondent, however, felt that verbal language should not be ignored: 'Arts therapists can sometimes be threatened by the verbal aspects and I think in that devalue the use of language. I think as arts therapists it's still important to be aware of the language we're using and the dynamics that are part of that language.'

Valikhani sees verbal therapy as a 'very Western concept' (2000: 86) and Wertheim-Cahen believes that 'the spoken word can only partly represent human experience, human expression and communication' (2000: 78). Dokter, however, notes that 'non-verbal communication is as culturally specific as verbal communication' (2000: 10). Music therapists Orth and Verburgt perhaps synthesize these perspectives, observing: 'It is a great advantage that there is no need to speak each other's language in order to listen to or make music. However, this does not mean the language barrier does not play a big role' (1998: 89).

The interviewees could be said to have identified a tension between the arts as language and language itself, through the varying perspectives they offer.

Theme 2: The importance of being understood/negotiating meaning

The importance of negotiating shared understanding with their clients, as bilingual dramatherapists working in an additional language, was discussed by all interviewees: 'I would explain at the beginning of the session that English was not my first language in case there are problems with understanding. It often changed a lot because I owned this.'

This implicit co-creation of meaning can have an impact on the therapeutic relationship, and highlights differing cultural ways of viewing the role of the therapist: 'When I don't understand a word I say so. This is levelling as there is an elevated view of the therapist in my country.'

Furthermore, the therapist's openness about working in an additional language was seen as an enabling factor in the process of facilitating understanding: 'It's important to say it so that an understanding of language becomes more negotiable'.

However, emphasis on the therapist's background could diminish the experience of the clients: 'I'm a foreigner too, can be disowning'. This disowning of difference suggests that if a therapist lays claim to a similar experience to that of the client, it could perhaps result in a feeling that the client's unique experience is somehow diminished.

Even when client and therapist share the same language, it may be important to negotiate meaning – 'There can be an assumption of similarity that doesn't necessarily exist' – which could lead to a client finding it hard to communicate authentically with the therapist or, as suggested above, that their own experience is unacknowledged or undervalued.

One dramatherapist emphasized the importance of checking the way something is understood by patients/clients: 'From my particular perspective as a foreigner, if you say something like this, I understand it like that. Is that what you're meaning to convey?'

This process of checking understanding could support a client in articulating their own experience, expressing and exploring their distinct identity. This raises the question of whether it is possible to be fully understood: 'Maybe not understanding and not being understood have to be part of the discourse when you're not sharing a language'.

Culturally specific meanings to words lead to dangers of misinterpretation – 'a house in English leads to a different image of the same subject in an Aboriginal language.' Sensitive exploration and acknowledgement of language differentials, along with careful negotiation of meaning, are seen by respondents as significant in the development of the therapeutic alliance.

Theme 3: The challenges of working with interpreters

Three respondents perceived working with interpreters as a potentially complicated and challenging area. The centrality of the arts as a form of communication was again suggested: 'It's tricky to have interpreter, the work loses immediacy. I try to rely on using the art form.'

The potential impact on the dramatherapy process itself was raised: 'It may change everything. It's a very grey area. A third person between the therapist and the client. Some issues may disappear.'

For instance, interpreters may live within the same community as the client, which can lead to difficulties that include a sense of divided loyalties, particularly in sensitive areas such as child abuse or self-harm. Gender, too, can sometimes present challenges: 'One difficulty could be gender. Arriving to see a client for the first time . . . a young man, opening the door to two women behaved in a way that the interpreter experienced as insulting. We needed to negotiate what felt feasible in working together. In the end a different interpreter was found.'

Several strategies were suggested for working effectively with interpreters. One therapist, for instance, had found it helpful to meet the interpreter before and after sessions. The debriefing was particularly important 'because the material often evoked stuff for the interpreter too'. The importance of ensuring the client was comfortable with the interpreter was discussed, illustrated by the following example from practice: 'Interpreters who can translate meaning rather than just words, so when I say "this", a person may understand it like "that". Is that what you mean? That is absolutely invaluable. And also incorporating at times some of the interpreters' suggestions too.'

This emphasizes the complex challenges of the interpreter's task. The importance of including interpreters in the process where relevant is further explained below:

> A male interpreter . . . had been a refugee himself, and quite aware of some of the clashes he experienced, and also other young men experienced culturally. He at times would say to me, "I've experienced this. Is it ok if I share that?"

Several respondents commented on the importance and complexity of the relationship between language and culture: 'Language isn't just a tool . . . it's an aspect of culture. Sometimes I found it more challenging, the cultural rather than the language differences.'

The interpreter, therefore, can be seen as a translator of culture, not simply of words. This perhaps illustrates the importance of checking the backgrounds of interpreters and clients, in case they have roots in different, even competing, cultures despite sharing the same or a similar language.

The use of interpreters is therefore viewed as an area of considerable complexity. One interviewee emphasized the importance of the interpreter being seen as a person in their own right, 'rather than just a mouthpiece, someone who was actually present in their own way' and as an interpreter of 'cultural meaning'. Dramatherapist, Dokter comments: 'The use of interpreters is not without complications in the area of client confidentiality and the need to interpret cultural assumptions underlying the language' (1998: 15). Further, political nuances of which the therapist is unaware, may be additional factors; Glenn notes that clients 'may be very worried that the interpreter belongs to a particular political faction within the community, which could lead to them being placed in danger' (2002: 183). This suggests a need to explore the position of an interpreter within the community for which they are translating, in case existing relationships are compromised and confidentiality threatened. Dokter notes that:

> Where clients bring discrimination and injustice, the experience of the interpreter may come to play a role in the session. The fact that in a more rural area where not many interpreters may be available, the same interpreter may be available in the therapy session, social service encounters and immigration interviews, needs to be considered. The interpreter can become a closer ally than the therapist in the practical arena.
>
> (Dokter 2000: 12)

Theme 4: Power issues/feeling disempowered

The impact of the therapist working in an additional language on the sense of personal and professional empowerment was a theme for three interviewees. One dramatherapist felt that language was used as a way in which the clients could 'get at her', particularly if dramatherapy was compulsory: 'My vocabulary was limited and the adults with learning disabilities would correct me'. This was explored in supervision and seen as a possible resistance mechanism: 'It was a challenge not to take it personally'.

Three dramatherapists referred to a sense of feeling inadequate at times, when working in a second language, regardless of their levels of fluency:

> Clinically experienced, I went into a situation where I felt very disempowered, deskilled . . . lack of confidence in the language affected me profoundly in terms of my skill-base. I know I have a whole body of experience. But that seemed to get very undermined in a sense, by feeling at times quite inadequate in terms of my capacity to communicate in words as fully as I might.
>
> (Dramatherapist A)

> I was a therapist for native English speakers who sometimes questioned my English. One client would ask in a patronizing manner if I had understood him.
>
> (Dramatherapist B)

When using stories, I need to spend more time preparing – to learn the vocabulary of the story as well as the story itself. This sometimes affects my confidence in telling it, especially if the story is relatively new to me but it also curtails, sometimes, the spontaneity of getting a flash of a similar story in a session and using it in the moment.

(Dramatherapist C)

Reflections were made about one dramatherapist's need to 'apologize' for her 'mistakes'. 'Why do I feel the need to do that? Am I apologizing for myself? Does it have to do with my resistances regarding my identity and learning the language properly? Why do I highlight the fact I make mistakes instead of just letting the mistakes happen, and deal with it in the moment if need be? Is this aspect of my persona having an adverse effect on my role as a therapist? This is an ongoing exploration, the roots of which I suspect lie in issues of identity and belonging.'

A lack of confidence in the majority language, however, enabled one therapist to develop sensitive attunement to the needs of the group in other ways, drawing more heavily on 'the process.' This theme was echoed by a dramatherapist whose first experience of working with an interpreter was utilizing sign language with a group with hearing loss, who reflected that it required 'an awareness of pace, body language and posture, enabling other people to lip-read if possible. Quite good training for working with interpreters of other languages.'

2 Reflections on respondents' own experiences as bilingual clients in therapy

As British dramatherapists are required to undertake therapy themselves during their training, this section will first explore their own experiences as clients working in an additional language. The following main themes were identified:

Theme 1:   The relationship between language issues and the therapeutic process.
Theme 2:   The importance of understanding and negotiating meaning.
Theme 3:   The use of mother tongue (L1) within therapy and the significance of being understood.

Theme 1: The relationship between language issues and the therapeutic process

Linguistic research has explored whether perhaps different 'selves' exist in different languages. Pavlenko suggests: 'Studies in psychoanalysis, psychology and linguistic anthropology demonstrate that bicultural bilinguals may exhibit different verbal behaviors in their two languages . . . may be linked to different linguistic repertoires, cultural scripts, frames of expectation, autobiographic memories and emotionality' (2006: 27). This suggests that access to different linguistic repertoires may be significant in the therapeutic process.

Indeed, one interviewee reflected that their experience of being a client in a second language may have been liberating: 'In my second language, I can be more direct than in my first language, so the fact they couldn't necessarily understand meant I did have permission to be more direct in my first language too'.

However, another interviewee spoke powerfully about their sense of disorientation: 'I wasn't fluent. The group were always changing between two languages. I felt alienated because I didn't really know what was happening. There would always be a sense of not feeling fully included.'

This respondent reflected that a sense of not being included, of feeling like an 'outsider', were powerful themes in their own therapeutic process. Further, that possibly the intense feelings of alienation triggered by language difficulties may have made it more possible to work on these issues in personal therapy.

Some psychoanalytical literature accords the concept of 'splitting' with particular relevance to people who are bilingual: 'We refer to the process of splitting the self from difficult emotions and experiences in order to defend from pain. This can serve a protective function or it can result in a distorted view and disconnection from self and others' (Dewaele and Costa 2013: 21). Different linguistic repertoires can contain 'different' selves. Therapeutic opportunities to integrate these 'selves' are further discussed in the closing reflections of this chapter.

Theme 2: The importance of understanding and negotiating meaning

The frustration of the struggle to be understood as a client was articulated by several therapists:

> 'Although fortunately I wasn't the only one in the group who had English as a second language . . . it helped not being the only one struggling with it, I wasn't used to speaking it on a daily basis . . . actually having to literally stamp the floor saying, "slower, I can't understand," but also finding that my peers would adjust to that.

Alternative means of expression, other than verbal, were drawn upon:

> I felt at times quite agitated about whether I would be understood and whether I could really express myself in a way adequately. I had to somehow find other ways of expressing myself and I think there was a lot

more gesticulation and expressing myself with my body . . . And the tone of my voice would change and somehow . . . it's very hard to put this into words . . . I had to just go to the absolute essentials of what I wanted to say.

This understandable frustration is echoed in Dewaele and Costa's research with migrants about their experiences in healthcare: 'They indicated that healthcare providers underestimated their language issues and that language barriers resulted in greater feelings of paranoia and aggression during their encounters with health providers' (2013: 20).

Theme 3: The use of mother tongue (l1) within therapy and the significance of being understood

The depth of their connection to their mother tongue was vividly explored by four respondents. They discussed feeling 'closer' to themselves, suggesting a transpersonal element to the connection: 'I felt more myself when I was speaking L1. It was closer to my soul.'

One therapist reflected that the mother is already communicating with the child as a foetus and that it is usually the mother who starts the communication process, commenting that even hearing another person speaking English in the same accent as her mother, triggered 'a sense of connection'. Another, however, who longed to communicate in L1 outside the therapy room, felt so profoundly accepted that she did not have the impulse to draw upon her mother tongue: 'The individual therapist gave me such a sense of acceptance of all that I was, that I didn't feel a lack of something.'

While research quoted here suggests that the opportunity to participate in therapy using one's mother tongue can be freeing, Casement is cited as giving the example of Samuel Beckett's choice to write in French, his second language: 'The only expedient by which he could gain his internal freedom and chances for creativity was, in Casement's opinion, the repudiation not only of his mother and motherland, but also and above all, of his mother tongue' (Dewaele and Costa 2013: 21). This echoes an earlier interviewee's comment that using a second language perhaps enabled them to access different aspects of themselves.

One respondent emphasized the importance of using L1 and of the other members of the group understanding their work: 'If I worked in L1, I did want to later explain to them, what they may not have understood.'

Several interviewees referred to the importance of working in L1, when exploring themes from early childhood that would have taken place in that language: 'And my therapist also would enable me if there were certain things that really pertained to my childhood, to be able to work in my own language. The others didn't necessarily understand.'

One therapist remembered reverting to L1 when expressing strong feelings: 'When expressing emotions I would revert to my first language, my mother tongue. Freeing.'

Is the mother tongue, therefore, the language of deeper emotion? There is some evidence for this: 'Bilinguals may perceive a first language to be more emotionally evocative because words and phrases in the first language are linked to emotionally relevant personal memories' (Harris, Gleason & Aycicegi 2006: 271). Indeed, several respondents alluded to their own need as clients to work in L1 to explore themes from early childhood. However, it is also suggested by Harris *et al.* that intense emotionality can also develop in a second language, as words and phrases in their second language become linked to emotional memories (Harris, Gleason & Aycicegi 2006).

3 Reflections on their work with bilingual clients

Having reflected on their experiences as bilingual dramatherapists, as bilingual clients as therapists themselves, the dramatherapists were now invited to discuss the implications for their work with bilingual clients. Similar themes emerged, indeed comments on the third theme echoed so closely the thoughts of the clients themselves that they have not been included here.

Theme 1: Language, power and cultural issues.
Theme 2: The use of mother tongue (L1) within therapy and the significance of being understood.
Theme 3: The importance of understanding and negotiating meaning.

Theme 1: Language, power and cultural issues

Two respondents discussed whether bilingual clients may sometimes be more comfortable working with bilingual dramatherapists. One mentioned having been sought out by a client who shared the same mother tongue. This could, however, bring its own challenges, as there could be 'an initial assumption about shared understanding which then had to be much more explicitly negotiated . . . where some of the differences in experiences were too'.

Two interviewees spoke about the impact of history and politics on the cultural and linguistic identity of the dramatherapist and client. One therapist, who comes from a European country with a considerable colonial history, commented:

I do accept that being taken as a representative of a colonial power with some of the responsibilities that are ascribed to people from that colonial power, both in terms of what has been inflicted in the past and what still continues to be played out now. By disowning it, it can't be worked with.

A second interviewee, who came from a formerly occupied country with a long history of oppression, talked about a client from Northern Ireland who particularly, given that she was living in Britain, did not want to want to work with a British therapist:

> Somebody told her: "what are you complaining about, because many experienced something similar". It was a therapist who told her this. She looked at this from a historical and cultural viewpoint. She added that she was aware that the therapist's home country had also experienced oppression.

The theme of uncertainty and lack of choice that can face migrants was discussed, referring to the example of an

> Iraqi Kurdish client who had to struggle with not being allowed to speak his language in school, having to learn Arabic, really struggling with the two languages, struggling with acquiring now a third language, English, in a context he hadn't chosen to learn. That whole area of difference and whether that implied differences of status he was very sensitive to. He could choose to go high or low status as the case might be. I had similar choices. As a therapist I had high status. As a woman, . . . I had fairly low status.

One context was also described in which all participants were bilingual, and the two languages were of roughly equal status: 'They were speaking both languages, swapping mid-sentence which was sometimes a bit confusing. There was a richness of language. Two vocabularies to draw on.'

The balance or imbalance of power described above is perhaps addressed by the interviewees' emphasis, cited earlier, on the importance of being understood, of acknowledging the fact that therapist and/or client are operating in an additional language and of engaging in a process of negotiated meaning. The co-creation of a strong therapeutic alliance is therefore arguably more complex in a multilingual context.

Theme 2: The use of mother tongue (II) within therapy and the significance of being understood

Two dramatherapists felt strongly that clients should be offered opportunities to work in L1. One considered that it may be important, while two therapists did not express their thoughts about this subject:

> Language – our emotional connection to groups, culture.

> Language is more than just spoken word and how we communicate. It represents some deeper heritage.

I feel in a therapeutic context the client feeling they have access to use their own language is terribly important.

One therapist felt that it was also important to learn some phrases in the language of the clients:

> Permission to use their own language, as well as finding ways to translate. I certainly have been known to work with dictionaries, both ways. Because that's always been important too, that it isn't just people having to communicate on my terms, that I also make the effort to try and communicate, where possible, in their language, even if it's just picking up a few core terms.

One dramatherapist wondered how it would be possible to work in L1 if the client would not be understood, but added: 'Where there is a sense of security, one can speak his own language. Maybe it wouldn't matter that no-one understands it. It's what it means to you.'

A study of work in the mother tongue and cultural matching in intercultural therapy emphasizes the importance of the solidity of the therapeutic alliance, reflecting that by offering the client the opportunity to work in L1 with a therapist who understood the language, 'the only way to reach him was to allow him to reach me, to see him in his totality, to hear his views, his side of the story and to stand next to him looking at the world' (2002: 53). This work, conducted in Urdu, perhaps suggests a kind of levelling, as the patient is communicating in the mother tongue and is understood by the therapist.

Concluding summary of main findings

The differences in views and experiences are perhaps as significant as the similarities. Respondents note the importance of negotiating meaning and checking understanding with clients, at the same time suggesting that the role of the therapist could be to support people in developing the resilience to cope with not being understood. The use of the mother tongue and/or additional languages in dramatherapy is viewed as more or less helpful at different times and for different reasons. The use of L1 is also perceived as important to some clients but not to others. Language differences are seen as having the potential to both impede and support mental health needs. Some bilingual clients find it enabling to work with bilingual therapists, whereas for others it is not a significant factor. For some, the cultural and linguistic backgrounds of therapist, client and interpreter are key factors to consider. The importance of exploring in depth the complexities of whether and how to work with interpreters was also a significant factor for bilingual dramatherapists and their clients.

The strength of feeling of two of the therapists' sense of disempowerment when facilitating dramatherapy in an additional language is of note, not just in terms of the particular power dynamics that may be at play in multilingual therapy, but in what it may indicate about a parallel process occurring for bilingual clients. Dewaele and Costa's study of beliefs, attitudes and practices of monolingual and multilingual therapists with their multilingual patients indicates that 'patients may feel distressed as a result of unacknowledged language proficiency differentials between patient and therapist' (2013: 20). Several felt that it was crucially important to offer bilingual clients the chance to communicate in L1. Others were less sure about the issue.

Power issues and the ensuing dynamics are compellingly discussed. Conci (2010) views psychoanalysis as presenting an opportunity for the healing of psychological and linguistic splits. He offered psychoanalysis to Italian migrants in Germany, in their mother tongue. He comments, 'my experience works in the direction of helping patients to maintain their Italian identity, feel at home in Germany and/or develop what we can call "a new German identity", and – last but not least – achieve a better integration between these two such diverse self-experiences and worldviews' (Conci 2010: 99). Further, Conci cites Kogan as seeing psychoanalysis as offering the possibility for integration of the two selves that may have emerged through operating in diverse cultures and languages: 'It was possible to bring the two self-representations together and to heal the psychic wound produced by migration' (2010: 107).

Strengths and limitations of the study

This research gives 'snapshots' of the experiences of five bilingual drama-therapists and their work with bilingual clients. Its strength lies in the richness of material, as well as the many years of collective experience represented. It brings together literature from the fields of psychoanalysis, psychotherapy, education, the arts therapies and dramatherapy, but omits texts from outside Europe, as well as those published in languages other than English. Further limitations include the omission of the specific contexts of the work and of the cultural and linguistic backgrounds of the therapists, in the interests of anonymity as well as the fact that it is not possible to generalize from the findings. Attempts have been made to diminish the effects of researcher bias through a reflexive approach, as well as affording the respondents the opportunity to check and amend material. Two therapists contacted me after the interviews, adding further points to their initial reflections, commenting how important it had been to have an opportunity to think about bilingual and multilingual dramatherapy, as well as their own experiences as bilingual therapists and clients.

Dramatherapy in the UK is still young in its research into bilingual contexts. However, it is hoped that the examples cited from the related literature can be applied to a dramatherapeutic context, albeit without drawing on the particular art form.

The interviews elicited rich data and while, as already stated, no general-izations can be made, the breadth and depth of experience represented, is considerable.

Recommendations

The interviews and literature pose a number of challenges for the profession. The interviews illustrate the complexity of linguistic and cultural identity and suggest that a range of issues require serious consideration in the interests of clients. While this study focuses on bilingual clients, it is probable that good practice in terms of language would be of benefit to all clients, regardless of linguistic background. For this reason, I have omitted the term 'bilingual' from some of the suggestions below. Recommendations for practice and research which emerge from this study, include:

1   an exploration of the therapeutic implications of language and cultural backgrounds of dramatherapists and clients within supervision and in training institutions;
2   for dramatherapists to consider checking any assumptions they may hold about language or languages spoken with the clients themselves and to engage with them in exploring which language they may prefer to work in;
3   to explore ways of negotiating meaning and understanding with clients;
4   to look at the implications of being and not being understood literally, metaphorically and therapeutically;
5   for professional associations to develop guidelines for good practice when working with interpreters;
6   for supervision and dramatherapy training institutions to explore, with dramatherapists and supervisors, the potential therapeutic impact of the dynamics of the language and cultural backgrounds of therapist, client and interpreters, from a range of perspectives that may include concepts such as 'splitting' and 'integration'; and
7   for further qualitative and quantitative research into bilingualism and dramatherapy.

It is hoped that this study will fuel further research into dramatherapy with bilingual practitioners and clients, as well as encouraging dramatherapists, supervisors and training institutions to further consider the psychological and therapeutic implications of bilingualism and the opportunities and challenges it can present. One dramatherapist commented after the interview, 'I am be-coming increasingly aware that when you by and large spend the majority of your days communicating in a second language, i.e., not your mother tongue, it is like a bereavement which is cultural and linguistic and which has a profound bearing on your sense of identity'. The respondents within this study offer a way forward with their insights into bilingualism, as well as practical examples of ways they have managed dramatherapy within bilingual and multilingual contexts.

Bibliography

Ball, J. (2011), *Enhancing Learning of Children from Diverse Backgrounds*, Paris: UNESCO.

Bhatt, S. (2013), 'Search for my Tongue', in *Collected Poems*, Manchester: Carcanet.

Blackwell, D. (2005), *Counselling and Psychotherapy with Refugees*, London and Philadelphia: Jessica Kingsley.

Braithwaite, T. (1998), 'Intercultural Dance, Theatre and Music as Facilitators in Creative Arts Therapy: A metacognitive experience', in D. Dokter (ed.) *Arts Therapists, Refugees and Migrants: reaching across borders* (pp. 191–205), London and Philadelphia: Jessica Kingsley.

Callary, B., Rathwell, S. & Young, B.W. (2015), 'Insights on the process of using interpretative phenomenological analysis in a sport coaching research project', *The Qualitative Report*, 20 (2) Article 1: 63–75.

Conci, M. (2010), 'An Advantage of Globalisation: Working with Italian patients abroad in their mother language', *International Forum of Psychoanalysis*, 19: 98–109.

Cresswell, J. (2007), *Qualitative Inquiry and Research Design*, Thousand Oaks, CA: Sage.

Cummins, J. (2001), 'Bilingual Children's Mother Tongue: Why is it important for education?' *Sprogforum*, 19: 15–20.

Dewaele, Jean-Marc and Costa, B. (2013), 'Multilingual clients experience of psychotherapy', *Language and Psychoanalysis*, 2 (2): 31–50.

Dokter, D. (ed.) (1998), *Arts Therapists, Refugees and Migrants: Reaching across borders*, London and Philadelphia: Jessica Kingsley.

Dokter, D. (ed.) (2000), *Exile: Refugees and the arts therapies*, Hatfield: Faculty of Art and Design, University of Hertfordshire.

Frie, R. (2013), 'Culture and language: bilingualism in the German-Jewish experience and across contexts', *Clinical Social Work Journal*, 41 (1): 11–19.

Gil, E. & Drewes, A. (eds.) (2005), *Cultural Issues in Play Therapy*, London and New York: Guilford.

Glenn, C. (2002), '"We Have to Blame Ourselves" – refugees and the politics of systemic practice', in R.K. Papadopoulos (ed.) *Therapeutic Care for Refugees: No place like home* (pp. 167–188), London: Karnak.

Harris, C.L., Gleason, J.B. & Aycicegi, A. (2006) 'When is a First Language More Emotional? Psychophysiological evidence from bilingual speakers', in A. Pavlenko (ed.) *Bilingual Minds: emotional experience, expression and representation* (pp. 257–283), Clevedon: Multilingual Matters.

James, J. (1998), 'Remembering: Intercultural Issues in integrative arts psychotherapy', in D. Dokter (ed.) (1998) *Arts Therapists, Refugees and Migrants: Reaching across borders* (pp. 206–16), London and Philadelphia: Jessica Kingsley.

Krause, I. (1998), *Therapy Across Culture*, London: Sage.

Li, W. (2000), *The Bilingualism Reader*, London: Routledge.

Mills, J. (2004), 'Mothers and Mother Tongue: Perspectives on self construction by mothers of Pakistani heritage', in A. Pavlenko & A. Blackledge (eds.) *Negotiation of Identities in Multilingual Contexts* (pp. 161–91), Clevedon: Multilingual Matters.

Moodley, R. & Palmer, S. (eds.) (2006), *Race Culture and Psychotherapy: Critical perspectives in multicultural practice*, London and New York: Routledge.

Orth, J. & Verburgt, J. (1998), 'One Step Beyond: music therapy with traumatised refugees in a psychiatric clinic', in D. Dokter (ed.) *Arts Therapists, Refugees and Migrants: Reaching across borders* (pp. 80–93), London and Philadelphia: Jessica Kingsley.

Pavlenko, A. (2006), 'Bilingual Selves', in A. Pavlenko (ed.) *Bilingual Minds: Emotional experience, expression and representation* (pp. 1–33), Clevedon: Multilingual Matters.

Skutnabb-Kangas, T. (1981), *Bilingualism or Not: The education of minorities*, Clevedon: Multilingual Matters.

Smith, J., Jarman, M. & Osborn, M. (1999), 'Doing Interpretative Phenomenological Analysis', in M. Murray & K.Chamberlain (eds.) *Qualitative Health Psychology* (pp. 218–40), Thousand Oaks, CA: Sage.

Valikhani, A (2000), 'Male Adults and Adolescents in Creative Art Therapy', in D. Dokter, (ed.) *Exile: Refugees and the arts therapies*, Hatfield: Faculty of Art and Design, University of Hertfordshire.

Wertheim-Cahen, T. (2000), 'What Options Does Art Therapy Offer for the Problems of Asylum Seekers', in D. Dokter (ed.) *Exile: Refugees and the arts therapies*, Hatfield: Faculty of Art and Design, University of Hertfordshire.

Zografou, L. (2012), 'The gifts of research – playing with phenomenology', *Dramatherapy, Official Journal of the British Association of Dramatherapists*, 34 (2): 83–91.

Chapter 3

Touching insights

Visual and tactile cultures in researching art psychotherapy with congenitally blind children

Uwe Herrmann

Introduction

My research as an art therapist in a German state school for the blind for 25 years grew from a necessity to understand the aesthetic and psychodynamic intricacies of this work, which caused me to embark on an extensive research journey. Drawing on case material from a cohort of four blind clients in long-term art psychotherapy, this research explored how blindness and sight engender gazes specific to the sensory differences between clients and therapist[1]. It explores how collaborative research with my blind clients led us to devise visual and tactile inquiry methods that considered our distinct sensory cultures, revealing the very psychodynamics between the sighted and the blind that I had set out to investigate.

Literature review: psychotherapeutic and psychological perspectives on blindness

Over decades researchers have noted the high occurrence of psychological disorders in blind children and agree that their ego development is considerably delayed due to the effect of sensory impairment on intersubjectivity between blind child and sighted parent (Adelson & Fraiberg 1973, 1974, 1976; Burlingham 1961, 1979; Curson 1979; Fraiberg 1968, 1977, 1979; Fraiberg & Freedman 1964; Klein 1962; Sandler 1965; Sandler & Wills 1963; Wills 1965, 1970; Wilson 1994). More recently, Hobson and Bishop (2003) have further highlighted congenital blindness disturbing the relational patterns between blind child and sighted carers in play, imitation, emotive expression, communication and understanding the mental and emotional processes of others.

This can be fully appreciated when considering the moment when a third object enters the space between mother and *sighted* infant, bringing about the phenomenon of 'joint visual attention', which involves the mastery of several things: establishing another person's line of sight towards an object; and understanding that another person can determine our line of gaze in the same way and that we can guide someone else's gaze to an object of our own scrutiny.

In this referential triangle, pointing delineates one's line of sight to another person (Butterworth 1998; Butterworth & Cochran 1980; Butterworth & Jarrett 1991; D'Entremont, Hains & Muir 1997). As mother and sighted infant look together at a third object, this invites referential vocalizations and words. Butterworth (1998) points to numerous studies clarifying the importance of joint visual attention for speech development.

Subsequently, joint attention has been explored as an underlying *sine qua non* for understanding the triangular relationship in art therapy (Damarell 1999; Isserow 2008, 2013; Herrmann 2006, 2007, 2009, 2010).

A different picture emerges when the child is born blind. Blind infants and sighted parents may establish joint attention by means other than vision, but little evidence exists about how effective this is (Landau1997; Landau & Gleitman 1985). Preisler found only occasional traces of pointing in blind children, often unnoticed by sighted parents. Interestingly, the introduction of objects was seldom organized around the needs of the sighted 'parents and their blind child together' (1997: 75), thus offering little opportunity for *shared* feelings and connectedness. Preisler found that parents varied dramatically in their responsiveness to blind children: some parents hardly shared feelings, adopting an instructive communication style. These problems carried into school years, where many blind children remained isolated and developmentally delayed.

Fogel (1997) believes that many blind children's psychosocial disorders are grounded in a sensory communicative mismatch between blind child and sighted pedagogue, stressing that blind children often feel alienated in a 'superior' sighted culture. These observations pinpoint a conundrum for therapy with the blind: while acknowledging the developmental cost of congenital blindness, psychoanalytic and psychotherapeutic authors do not address the implications of the different sensory cultures of the sighted and the blind. Physical contact between client and therapist is – for ethical reasons – abstained from in therapy training and practice. Inferring this cultural etiquette from work with the sighted to the blind leaves language or sound as the main *shared* sensory modality for asserting presence, joint attention and communication; and it creates a one-sided situation where the patient is seen by the therapist but cannot see her or him in return. Psychotherapy as a 'talking cure' might be sufficiently applicable to the adolescent or adult blind patient accustomed to a non-touch interpersonal sighted culture. However, a physically abstinent model of therapy with the blind *child* creates a sensory gap, replaying the mismatch between different sensory cultures that Fogel described.

Thus, the particular psychodynamics between the blind client and sighted therapist, each part of a different sensory culture, remain unclear. What are the implications if a blind client experiences vision as something a sighted therapist can unilaterally 'do to' her or him? How does the young blind patient react to a therapist who refrains from touching and from being touched while simultaneously being capable of 'touching' the child by looking? This question of touch is even more prominent when art becomes part of the blind-sighted relationship, i.e. in art education and in art psychotherapy and, though not clarified, is nonetheless traceable in the literature.

Art education, art therapy and blindness

Though educationalists for the blind had continuously denigrated tactile aesthetics (Hayhoe 2008), the exceptional artist–educator Viktor Lowenfeld established, against considerable resistance, sculpture classes at Vienna's Jewish Institute for the Blind, until he was exiled to the USA in 1938 (Michael 1981, 1982; Saunders 1960, 2001). However, Lowenfeld did not investigate blind children's sculptures the same way he systemized sighted children's drawing development from scribble to symbol (Lowenfeld & Brittain 1957). Rather, all sculptures he describes begin *after* the onset of symbolism. This omission concerns the essential question how the blind child masters the transition from non-representational to symbolic artwork. It is here that the role of touch comes into play. Hayhoe (2005) points to the lack of case studies in Lowenfeld's writing, with one significant exception: his work with Camilla, an 11 year-old deaf–blind girl (Ulman 1987; Michael 1982). Camilla's parents had kept her hidden, chained and isolated. Upon her discovery the girl was taken to the Perkins Institute, where staff were unable to communicate with her. Called to help, Lowenfeld describes how gradually, by touched-based interpersonal contact and joint art-making, Camilla learned to symbolize and to talk. Revisiting this case reveals much that Lowenfeld left unstated: in a developmental order, Camilla seemed to arrive at symbolic, representational artwork *because* Lowenfeld relied on interpersonal touch, followed by pre-symbolic modelling, (self-)representational modelling and finally language. Lowenfeld's enormous tactile investment seems key to his success. We can clearly see how Lowenfeld fostered a culture of joint tactile attention, which, at the interface of education and therapy, resulted in the girl's psychological development.

Edith Kramer, another 1938 Viennese émigrée, pioneered art-therapy theory alongside her practice with blind children (1971, 1979, 2000). She ascribed a strengthened feeling of self in her blind clients to her key idea of sublimation through art-making in art therapy. Kramer did not discuss distinct sensory cultures when working with the blind, but the issue of touch is traceable. Kramer (1971, 2000) accounts how her enormous amount of physical and aesthetic assistance was helpful. She termed this ability as the 'Third Hand', which the art therapist lends to the client and which, other than the auxiliary ego, becomes physically and aesthetically manifest (Kramer 1986).

Similarly, Henley (1991, 1992) draws attention to the art therapist's highly active role in the blind child's exploration and awareness of the art materials and product; and Rubin (1976, 1978) researched blindness as the source of a distinct *tactile* aesthetics.

My own work with the blind resulted in a number of papers; I described the modifications of my therapeutic posture to accommodate the client's sensory impairment by interventions akin to Kramer's 'Third Hand' concept (Herrmann 2001). Researching body image development in a single-case study on a congenitally blind girl, I found that clay modelling facilitated her development of body image alongside her ego structures and self-reflection. Further, I identified two main agents in art therapy's efficacy in the case: modelling served as a repressive 'filter' due to its sensory qualities and the ensuing sculptures functioned as a 'tactile mirror' for body image formation (Herrmann 1997, 2011). In other papers I described how my blind clients and I gradually learned to place touch centre stage and worked towards joint *tactile* attention (Herrmann 1995, 1997, 2006, 2007, 2009, 2010).

The scarce literature on art therapy with the blind leaves much unexplored, i.e., the art therapist's role as a representative of the sighted culture and its implications for transference, art-making and reflection in therapy. Thus, the particular psychodynamics of art therapy with the blind in relation to touch, a joint sensory culture and the gaze experience remain unclear. It was from here that eventually the central question of my research grew: what is the nature of the gaze experience within the triangular relationship in art psychotherapy with the congenitally blind?

As this question was linked to my practice, this practice strongly determined my research methodology.

Methodology for data collection and analysis

Practice research requires methods that are useful to our question and manageable in the context of our work. My practice had involved 200 individual processes of several years each. I therefore created an archive, comprising past and current work, many thousands of session notes, photographs of clients' artwork, and audiotaped, transcribed retrospective review sessions held regularly upon ending therapy.

From this archive it transpired that my clients' diverse visual impairments and added disabilities potentially clouded the issue in which I was interested. Discussing the emerging figures with my supervisors, I decided to focus on congenital blindness to pinpoint my main question: how does the fact that a client is blind while the art therapist is sighted influence the dynamics of art psychotherapy?

Focusing on congenital blindness, the following inclusion and exclusion criteria were applied:

Exclusion: children continuing in therapy (as this would have impinged on the therapeutic relationship) and past clients (as retrospective permission might have been difficult to obtain).

Inclusion: children, whose leaving was imminent. Two girls and two boys met these criteria.

My first survey re-familiarized me with the entire body of my clinical material and influenced methodological considerations. Available records of individual art-therapy processes offered a wealth of information: they contained *stories*. This called for a narrative case-study approach, in which I could describe and analyse the clients' processes using case notes and the clients' artwork retrospectively. In addition, audio-recorded retrospective review sessions could involve my clients in the research to counterbalance my own ideas.

I could therefore draw from multiple sources and use a blend of methods sympathetic to the material, my research interest and my situation as a practitioner: case studies and visual methods i.e. the retrospective review and analysis of clients' images and a cautiously collaborative element.

Case study and case cohort

Narrative case studies describe and reflect practice; confirming, challenging, or modifying established theory, they are particularly suited to areas lacking an extensive knowledge base. They are determined by four factors: they provide *narrative*-knowing, analyse *complexity*, create *contextualized* knowledge and analytically describe *practical expertise* in action (McLeod 2010). Given the immediacy of my practice with the blind, and the paucity of specific literature, this method seemed to fit: I could unpack therapeutic processes while two supervisors would respond to the narratives and my discussion.

Thus, we might say that the closer the 'culture' of an inquiry's methods is to the 'culture' of its researched practice, the less alienating research feels to the practitioner. We might also say that while therapy helps to make sense of one's 'life's story', the same can be said for the narrative-knowing a case study induces; it establishes relationships between experiential fragments and systematically explains their underlying unconscious connections, only partially understood at the time of therapy.

This is particularly helpful considering the intricacies of therapy, which constantly shifts between past and present, the conscious and the unconscious, feeling and thinking. In art therapy, the making, aesthetic traits and meaning of patients' artwork increase this complexity: the patient–artist shifts between being maker, audience and interpreter of her or his artwork, the art therapist's role likewise shifting between observation, intervention and interpretation. This constitutes a complexity, which the case-study method's narrative and analytic procedures can encompass.

Gilroy (1992) stresses the role of the case study in art therapy as 'cumulative evidence'. Similarly, Edwards (1999) highlights its strengths by involving the client's, the therapist's and the supervisor's voice. McLeod (2001, 2010) points to examples of such rigorously analysed case narratives. All emphasize the importance of rigour in response to the critique that single-case studies have received: incomplete records; bias through retrospective adjustment of events and observations; absence of other opinions, i.e. the client's, on therapy's effectiveness; and lack of proof for systematic interpretation of the material. McLeod (2010) addresses these concerns with a 'battery' of strategies: including multiple data sources; thorough narrative of the therapeutic process and analysing change in relation to time; cross-comparison with other cases; critical examination of alternative interpretations; inclusion of the *clients'* perspective on their process and data analysis; serious consideration of theory for cross-case comparison; self-reflexivity and provision of information on the researcher's context to identify potential bias (McLeod 2010: 28).

Whereas single-case studies analyse the variance within one case, my research compared four individual long-term cases. What was the rationale behind researching several cases in conjunction? Single-case research has been critiqued for lacking in generalizability (McLeod 2010). A case cohort, however, compares several cases united by several shared characteristics, allowing for pattern recognition: we can see how individual experience is embedded within a larger picture (Creswell 2007; Yin 2009; Gilroy 2006; McLeod 2010). Similarities and discrepancies can emerge across cases, adding to the credibility of findings, as they occur in more than one individual.

Case cohorts combine the single-case's depth with a contextual cross-comparison, while small participant numbers prevent the researcher from becoming overwhelmed by the multitude of data generated by multiple sources. They have been previously used in art-therapy research (Wood 2002; Rehavia-Hanauer 2003; Damarell 2011).

Several factors made clients in my study cohere as a cohort: (1) congenital blindness; (2) age, i.e. from the onset of puberty to adolescence; (3) psychological distress manifested at school; (4) uninterrupted art-therapy processes that were about to terminate; and (5) long-term art therapy between four and six years.

Client collaboration

Narrative descriptive case studies are often told from the vantage point of the therapist, and McLeod (2010) has therefore advocated including the clients' thoughts in the study to objectify the researcher's ideas. Similarly, Gilroy (1992: 237) suggested that 'perhaps as researchers we should pay attention to the patient's assessment of a successful outcome in art therapy'. This conforms to collaborative research models in psychotherapy (Yalom & Elkin 1974; Mearns & Thorne 1988; Dryden & Yankura 1992) and has been demonstrated in art therapy by McClelland (1993), Dalley, Rifkind & Kim (1993), and Herrmann (1997, 2011).

However, client participation in research must consider the patient's vulnerability (Fox, Martin & Green 2007). In my study, I invited clients whose therapy was about to terminate to partake in audiotaped and transcribed retrospective review sessions upon ending therapy. This procedure guaranteed that clients would not see research as an unwarranted means to continue our relationship, and yet our recorded sessions contained their ideas. I explained to my clients how a review of our work would help us to see what had been achieved and that my research would help me learn about what art therapy at the school for the blind entailed. This learning aspect may be fully appreciated when seen in the context of the 'learning culture' it was embedded in: a school for the blind operated largely by sighted experts.

My clients' response was very encouraging: they greatly welcomed that I, as a sighted expert in an educational setting, was a learner of sorts, just as they were, and that my learning depended on their ideas. Client collaboration as a methodological choice lent expertise to the client, fostering a culture of mutual curiosity and expert knowledge.

Gilroy (2006: 100) outlines that researching a cohort in art therapy often includes 'visual methods to identify patterns and visualities' across cases. In my study, using such *visual* and *tactile* methodology proved beneficial and intrinsic: it took the issue of shared sensory culture(s) between therapist/researcher and client/researcher to the heart of the investigation.

Visual methods

Art-therapy practice makes us expert 'lookers' who engage with client's imagery visually before we verbalize its 'meanings'. This expertise, based on our visual faculties, can be a source for knowing. Gilroy (2006) observes how the analysis of imagery in art-therapy research is related to the traditions of art history, where visual artwork is described to an audience who cannot partake in the experience of looking at the real object. Sullivan (2010) suggests that David Hockney's (2001) expertise as an artist made him *look, observe, compare, think, draw on additional sources and theorize* to arrive at his conclusions when researching stylistic changes in historical European painting. Such visual processing allows looking to claim a place in research that was previously dominated by the verbal even when its subject was primarily visual. I will return to these art-based strategies of inquiry when I speak about the analysis of the clients' sculptures through visual and tactile displays.

Schaverien (1992, 1993, 1995) outlines the retrospective review of many images by individual clients in art therapy, offering new insights compared to earlier understandings in therapy. She illuminates how the visual analysis of artwork encompasses several strategies: systematically analysing the image's formal elements, i.e. the shapes, colour, and form of marks; documenting the changes in imagery over time; recording the therapeutic process and the patient's verbatim commentaries; and comparing the patient's experience or appraisal of the therapeutic process with that of the therapist.

In my research, handling and photographing artwork and visually presenting it for the present study was an engaging experience, involving me with the material on a sensory and aesthetic level.

Looking through the lens of the camera: visual thinking in practice

The extensive photographic record of my clients' artwork towards a visual archive became an exercise in thinking based on looking. This began at the point of seeing the work through the camera's lens and then carried into the subsequent processing of visual records. While I had perceived sculptures individually in therapy, they now started to cross-refer. I began to see and understand sculptural groups that 'stood out' by sharing formal qualities. These thoughts were 'visually based', i.e. 'here we have yet another one of these flat/round/oblong/marked/fractured things' or 'this figure's posture reminds me of others'. Such concept formation operated first within the 'closed entity' of each client, but eventually reached across cases when I re-immersed myself in the material.

As this happened prior to writing up and analysing the case narratives, visual-concept formation preceded and guided my verbal reflection. Such thinking, based on looking, happens in art therapy while we absorb the client's artwork visually and make sense of it in verbal thinking later. In research this can be done with the privilege of time and a complete view of the material, as opposed to a session's limited perspective. Sculptural groups would have been far more complicated to extrapolate from written notes without any preceding visual thinking. Therefore, documenting and visualizing the clients' artwork placed the artwork centrally to the investigation, bringing the culture of art-therapy practice and the culture of research to join forces.

As a preliminary impression, I gathered at the time that a considerable portion of clients' early artwork lacked in representational, symbolic concern. This had puzzled me in therapy and continued to do so during visual documentation. I also noted how representational sculptures appeared in individual clients' work mostly towards the later phases of therapy. Still, the implications of this observation were unclear.

Photographing the artwork catered to my visual predilections, and also made me think harder about me and my clients' sensory differences. Ironically, it was the visual nature inherent to this portion of my research that made me more aware of how a mutual, touch-based and largely unconscious culture had developed in therapy. Simultaneously, my handling of the sculptures for visual documentation deepened my tactile familiarization with the artwork. This, I suggest, replayed the larger, ongoing process underlying my clinical work with the blind: I, as a sighted person, had needed to 'recalibrate' in relation to *their* impairment to develop a shared sensory culture. The more I was drawn to other sensory modes rather than to vision, the more I could think about vision and blindness, and vice versa.

The intensity of touching and looking at the artwork made me rethink my research focus. I became aware of my visual hardwiring, and began to wonder about the gaze between congenitally blind clients, a sighted art therapist and the artwork: what was the fate of my gaze in this encounter? Was there a sort of 'gaze' that my congenitally blind clients carried to our sessions? Could the term extend to congenitally blind clients at all? From these thoughts the focus of my research emerged: investigating the *gaze* in art psychotherapy with the congenitally blind.

The studio collection: artefacts, curation and tactile culture

Documenting all past and present artwork I realized that sculptures left behind by clients had amounted to a vast collection, which, partly displayed in the studio, was available to my gaze and to my succeeding blind clients' touch: over years the art-therapy studio had grown into a space merging visual and tactile *cultures*.

I became aware of this collection's inherent 'legacy' and responsibilities; I had become a curator of sorts. Photographing the artwork revealed how active my counter-transference still was after my clients had left, as I gave a kind of care to their artwork that they often had felt lacking in their parents. In her essay *Dead Stock: The Researcher as Collector of Failed Goods,* Celeste Olalquiaga (2008) draws parallels between the cultures of research and collecting, and illuminates that particularly collections of the non-commercial kind represent a surplus, leftover or residue:

> Bereft of primary cultural value and/or circulation, the items . . . are no longer in use, and the pleasure they offer is derived in part from their inherent anachronism and/or marginalization, which renders them witness, or traces, of a different time. Displacing economic or aesthetic criteria, their main worth is often based on 'possession', or its imaginary experience.
> (Olalquiga 2008: 39)

The terms 'failed goods' and 'marginalization' are key when rethinking why I had gathered artwork by individuals from a marginalized group of people. Collecting their artwork I had unconsciously picked up on the dynamics that underpin the dilemma between sighted parents and blind children: seeing and not being seen, or overlooking and being overlooked. Safeguarding the work I had provided a container for the residue of 'failed' developmental experiences from which they needed to separate.

The collection included hundreds of pieces that seemed fragmented and meaningless in therapy. Discarding this artwork, or leaving it undocumented because of its 'poor' aesthetic quality or 'obviously insignificant meaning', might have hampered narrating clients' stories, constituting a particularly *sighted* bias and severely curtailing the study's question. My indiscriminate care for the entire artwork revealed three things: my hope that eventually comprehension would be born from comprehensiveness; that such work contained an element of our work still needing to be understood; and that this was possibly for blind and sighted aesthetic predilections, development and culture.

Tactile panoramic displays and visual tableaux

Preparing the individual retrospective review sessions, Schaverien's (1992) retrospective review of images had inspired me to build a tactile retrospective display of each client's artwork when ending therapy. I had arrayed the entirety of each client's artwork chronologically on the studio tables, with cards noting their beginning and completion, and explored these displays with each client individually.

I decided to facilitate these free-floating sessions with a very 'loose' range of questions to my client and myself: Do I remember sculpture? When was it made? What do I remember from this time? What was it called? How do I feel about it now? Does it relate to any other artwork? This was what would naturally happen upon ending therapy and therefore would not make me concentrate on my research interests to the neglect of any issues the clients might have.

These tactile displays reminded me of panoramas, each some ten to twenty metres long (Figure 3.1). Their chronological structure had an enormously 'ordering' effect on my own and my clients' recall of therapy. This made me think that we had mutually forgotten some 'fuzzy' part of their processes, particularly all clients' early, non-representational artwork, which I had found hard to understand in therapy.

The retrospective review sessions replayed these problems, but it was good to see this early work in sequence and to observe how meaning was still difficult to construe. Clients apparently recalled their later sculptures most easily and had considerably more to say about them. It emerged in the review that they had worked significantly longer on these sculptures, coinciding with a turning point in therapy and art-making that now seemed to surface as an easy 'recall'.

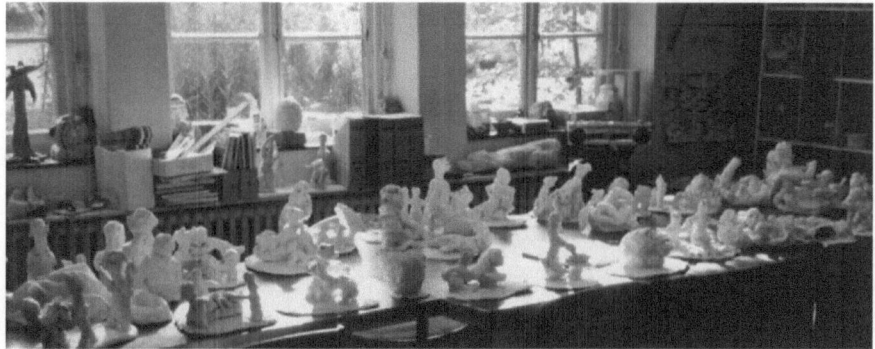

Figure 3.1 The tactile panoramic review session

The ensuing analysis of data revealed that this recall and understanding of sculptures corresponded to their degree of representational symbolisation and to my clients' ability to reflect and verbalize: early pre-symbolic sculptures, though numerous, were much harder to discuss than later symbolic ones.

In terms of a shared sensory culture, the retrospective reviews and panoramic displays replayed therapy in fast motion, revealing the enormous journey each client had ventured: laying down the foundations of making, looking, thinking and speaking, or, in other words, the foundations of joint attention, symbolization, mentalization, verbalization and reflection.

Exploring the sculptural panoramas, we identified significant experiences and interlocking thematic groups, enabling us to pinpoint key sculptures that would best represent a category as a core around which the other sculptures clustered. My clients' comments became a crucial source of data, assuming a prominent position in all the stages of the subsequent research process: our joint explorations took the lead in helping me to formulate my ideas, while my eyewitness records of their art process, together with my notes and their verbatim commentary, provided a rich context in which to analyse and interpret the artwork.

Having identified clusters and key sculptures from the tactile displays, I now needed to present the material for visual analysis, looking at how individual sculptures 'behaved visually' in context in order to understand their inter-relations. I created chronological tableaux of individual photographs showing the entirety of clients' art production, which provided an ordered, compact field for visual cross-referencing. From such overall tableaux, smaller 'sub-tableaux' could be extracted, uniting sculptures belonging to one group and making their connection visually apparent. Though this procedure picked up

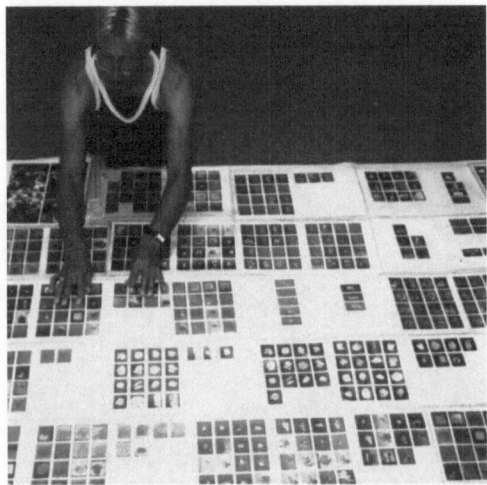

Figure 3.2 Producing the visual tableaux

on the tactile displays, its visual nature and aesthetics spoke to my sighted eye, while the panoramas had catered to my clients' blindness.

Ethical considerations and research design

Ethical considerations

When therapists investigate their own work the potential conflict of interest between the roles of practitioner and researcher must be considered (Ezzy 2002; Fox, Martin and Green 2007; Creswell 2009; McLeod 1994, 2010).

Gilroy (2006) points out that educational settings often lack guidelines for research. Though the management of the School for the Blind quickly approved of my inquiry, providing I followed the school's general data protection policy, I felt that I needed to augment these standards by four strategies:

1   reviewing the literature on ethics in therapy research
2   comparing my inquiry to existing procedures
3   providing expert consultation
4   putting the interest of my clients, as seen from my perspective as their *therapist*, paramount.

Reviewing the literature was helpful, and McLeod (2010) points to three main ethical concerns in case-study research: the client's informed consent; confidentiality; and avoiding harm to clients. I addressed the first two issues by devising contracts and consent forms, explaining in depth to my clients and their carers what research involved and how to withdraw, and how to contact the institution's verbal psychotherapist to discuss any issues arising from research with another person. I also explained that all material would be anonymized and kept confidential. These strategies were in tune with existing procedures described by the literature and by research experts I consulted.

The third issue, harm to patients, required further thought and consideration of my double perspective as practitioner–researcher. As McLeod (2010: 71) points out, harm can occur in multiple ways, and the time when clients are asked for participation is crucial to ensure that they are able to 'meaningfully say "no"'. I shared this concern and asked my clients at a point when therapy was 'naturally' ending. McLeod (2010: 65) has outlined that such late client participation may constitute a useful compromise, because it is grounded in an established relationship and less likely to impact the process.

This thinking met with my own as a therapist. When my clients started therapy participating in a research project was not in sight, and therefore I conducted the retrospective review sessions as usual and unrelated to my research question. Yet, the experience of collaborative research upon ending therapy constituted a cultural shift in therapy that was actually beneficial to patients' leaving process in a way I had not foreseen.

Research stages

In the following section I detail the research stages and how these early steps were situated within the inquiry's overall sequence.

Findings: how culture manifests in therapy and research

From the visual analysis of artwork, written case notes and retrospective review material three distinct forms of artwork emerged in a developmental order.

First, *protomorphous artwork*: pre-symbolic, non-representational, often fragmented and nameless forms that occurred early in therapy. These forms were mainly centred around the clients' tactile involvement and explorations, inviting little verbal discourse during therapy and in the review. Nonetheless,

Table 3.1 Research stages

Stage		Goal	Procedure
1	First survey	To identify all individual clients by age, diagnoses, and duration of stay	Written and statistical evaluation based on clients' records
2	Documentation	To document all individual clients' processes in art therapy from 1991 to current	Creation of a visual and written archive; photographing, dating and chronologically archiving clients' artwork Written lists of artwork noting date, session number, title and technique Word-processing case notes
3	Cohort selection	To define the study's focus	Selection of clients from the visual and written archive matched by congenital blindness, age, and uninterrupted stay in long-term art therapy
4	First immersion	To collaboratively identify key sculptures and groups by form and content	Creation of tactile panoramas of clients' sculptures; conduction of audiotaped retrospective review sessions; transcription of tapes
5	Second immersion	To understand and discern clients' sculptures visually	Creation of visual tableaux comprising overviews of all work and of sculpture groups based on similarities of form and content; visual thinking
6	Third immersion	To write up the case narratives	Looking at the entirety of the visual and text-based data Description of images and sessions in depth Thinking in words

continued

Table 3.1 continued

Stage		Goal	Procedure
7	Review of the historic literature on blindness	To establish the general background of the study	Reviewing the historic literature on pedagogy, psychoanalysis and psychotherapy, art and art therapy with the blind
8	Review of the literature on the 'gaze'	To establish the particular background of the study and the research questions	Reviewing the specific literature on the 'gaze' in art, philosophy, psychoanalysis, psychology, visual studies and art psychotherapy Formulating research questions
9	Categorization	To identify 'gaze' categories in the triangular relationship between blind client, artwork and sighted art therapist	Interrogating formal, thematic and relational elements in the case notes, artwork, and visual tableaux within each individual case
10	Phenomeno-logical reduction	To conceptualize recurring and significant examples of the gaze and to identify possible alternative ways of understanding	Re-interrogating case notes, artwork and visual tableaux and cross-comparing material from all four cases
11	Triangulation of emerging ideas	To further conceptualize and contextualize gaze categories with the clients' experience	Triangulating emerging ideas on the gaze with the clients' ideas on their process by using the retrospective review session transcripts
12	Interpretation of findings	To discuss and establish the findings in relation to theory	Discussing the findings against the backdrop of the reviewed literature

these forms seemed a fundamental step in artistic development, akin to sighted children's scribbles. This revealed that for most blind clients, unlike most sighted peers, art therapy had been their first and deepest exposure to art-making. This pre-symbolic work showed that art therapy provided clients with a long-needed, psychologically formative cultural experience at the earliest possible stage.

Second, *allomorphous artwork*: figurative, symbolic representations that carried meaning and were set in the middle phase of therapy. These forms comprised increased joint tactile involvement of client and therapist, and invited verbal discourse. Clients noticeably abstained from relating any of the figures' symbolic concern to themselves. Rather, they were related to an outside 'other'. This artwork dealt with the fundamental recognition that something 'other' could be symbolized, objectified, differentiated, talked about and reflected towards a mutual aesthetic culture based on touch, language and thought.

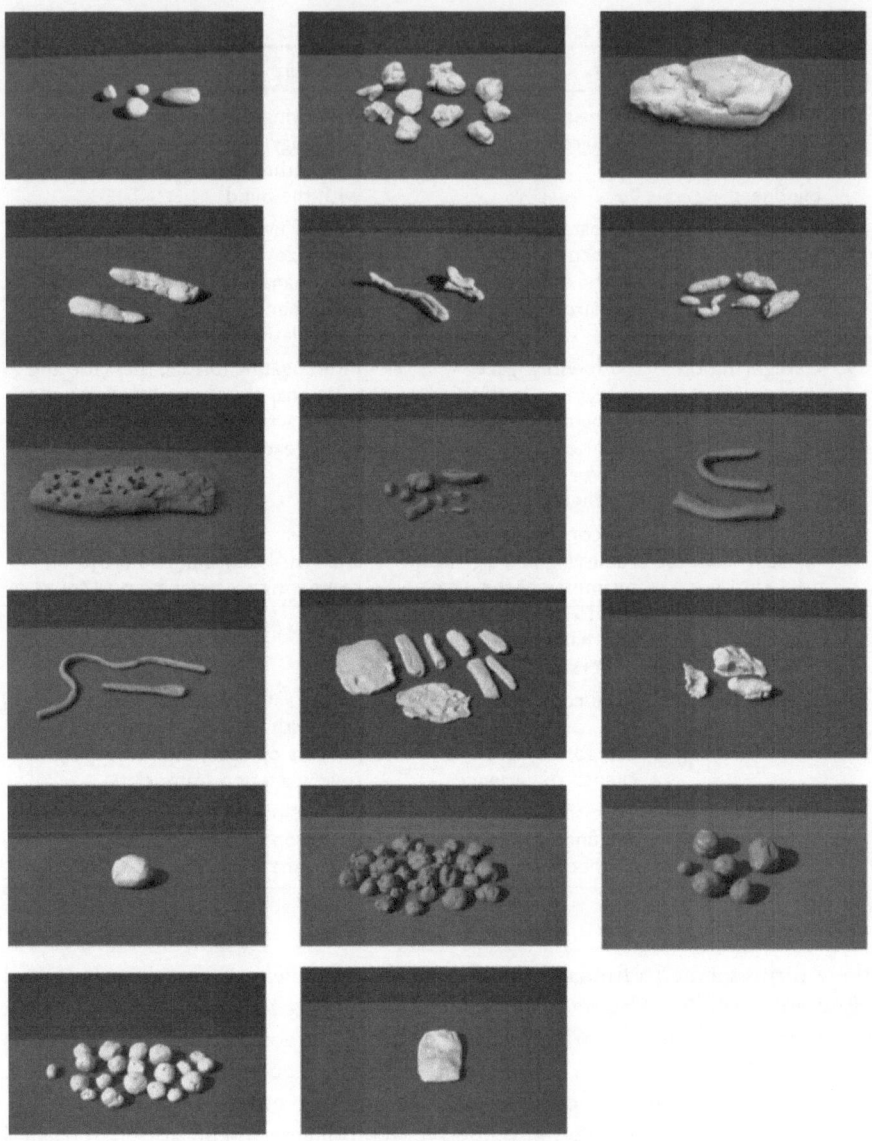

Figure 3.3 Protomorphous sculptures

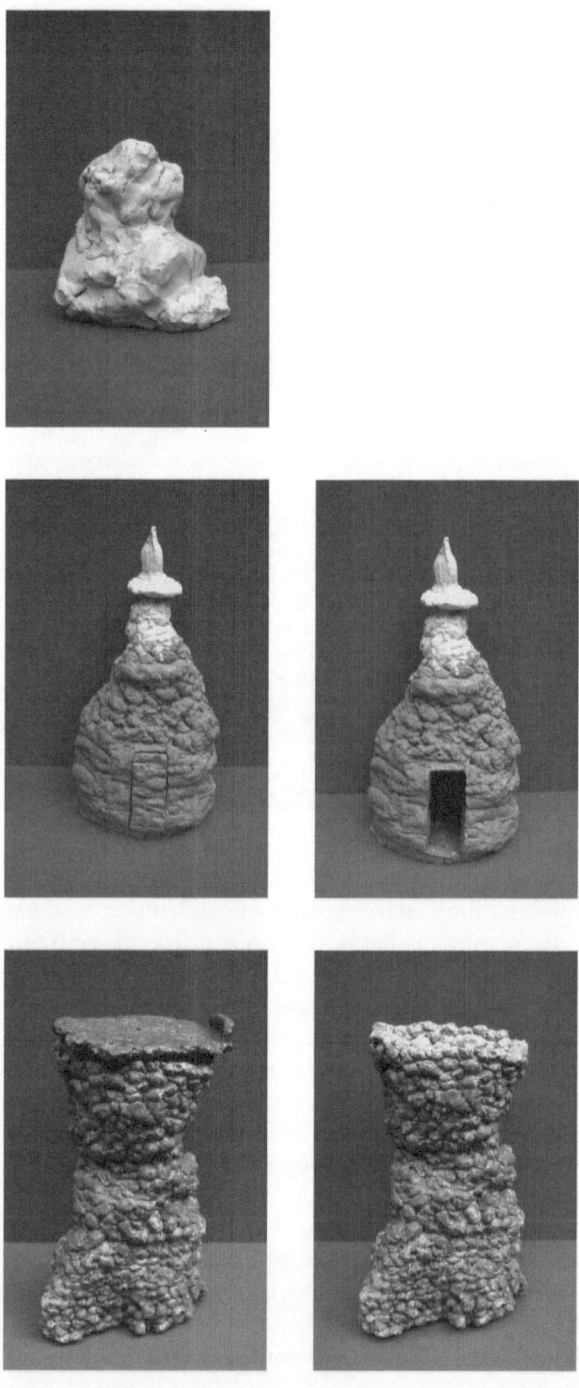

Figure 3.4 Allomorphous sculptures

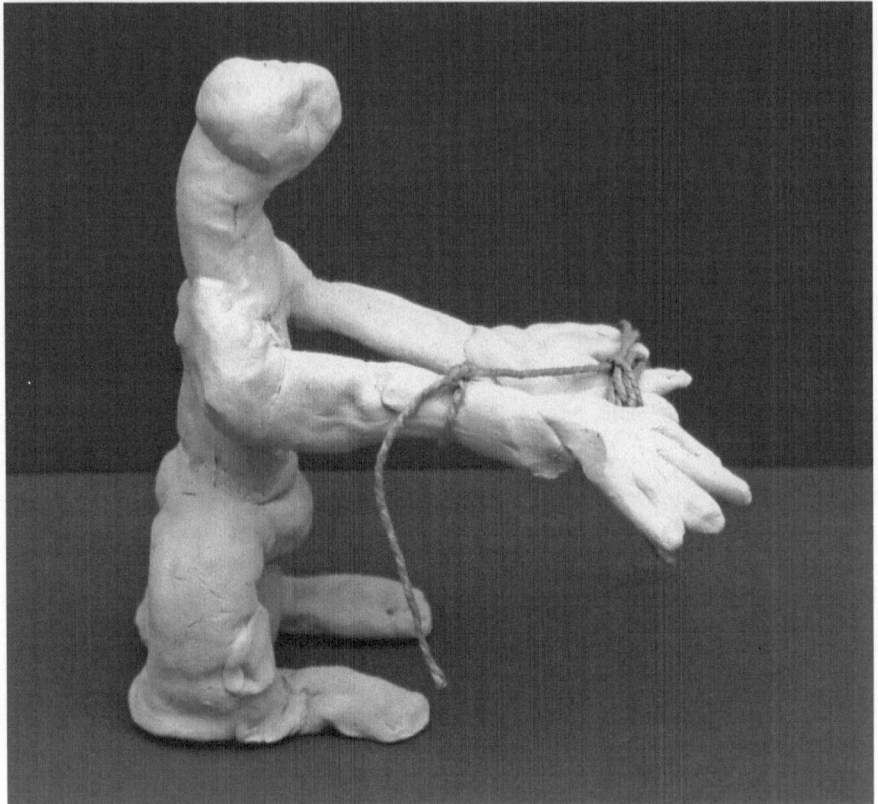

Figure 3.5 Automorphous sculpture

Third, *automorphous artwork*: symbolic self-representational sculptures, always set at the end of therapy, culminating in clients' denomination of these figures as a loveable, accepted image of their 'self'. These sculptures induced noticeably heightened joint tactile involvement of client and therapist, and a further increased verbal discourse. In this final group of artworks, often consisting of one decisive and unique sculpture, clients succeeded in giving up their formerly fused state and made themselves subject of joint aesthetic and verbal reflection.

Alongside a progressive increase in tactile joint attention and verbal activity, the occurrence of these three artwork categories engendered distinct gazes that gradually enhanced the clients' conscious reflection. These 'gazes' were:

A *protoreflective gaze*: the client's reflective activity was solely sensory, the art material providing a mirroring experience, which eschewed any reference to other persons or the self.

An *alloreflective gaze*: the client's reflective activity ventured towards the 'other', i.e. family, peers or the therapist.

An *autoreflective gaze*: the client's reflective activity was increasingly directed at their emotional and mental processes. They revisited their biographies and their relationship to the therapist on a higher level and, reaching a loving 'gaze' at themselves, finally decided that therapy was complete.

In other words, clients evolved a developmentally increasing reflective ability, of first the arts materials on a sensory level, then a reflection of 'other' in relation to 'self', finally arriving at a dynamic, changed and loveable self-image towards the end of therapy. Alongside the occurrence and development of distinct forms of artwork, the degree of joint attention, symbolization, mentalization and verbal reflection steadily increased, while psychologically disturbing symptoms and behaviour decreased.

Investigating the nature of the interpersonal gazes, the intricacies of transference, power and surveillance between blind client and sighted therapist emerged. Our respective gazes in therapy were subject to unconscious dynamics that mirrored the continued historic, cultural and psychological misunderstandings between the blind and the sighted:

The client's 'blind gaze' often demanded and yet frustrated my sighted visual gaze. My sighted, visual gaze initially often surfaced as an interpersonal sensory mismatch, unfruitful instructions or interventions, or lack of adequate interventions.

Beginning the inquiry, I had a rather vague idea of what I was looking for and what I would find, and I returned from research with much more than expected: the recognition of how and why practice with the blind engenders a changed sensory culture that can reconcile a fundamental perceptual divide. This shared culture crucially depends on mastering tactile joint attention and a 'tactile gaze'.

Reflections and conclusions

The thoughts emerging from this study have helped me develop my understanding as to how a blind client, especially a young blind child, is able to make use of the art materials, the therapeutic relationship and art therapy. The findings have provided me with a working model that can be applied and tested in daily practice, in determining how, when and why current clients' development changes and how I can be of better use to them. I became aware that my clients' change was matched by a fundamental change in my own therapeutic posture, my attitude to a shared sensory culture, issues of joint tactile attention and, alongside all these, the question of adequate, touch-based interventions.

Such thoughts may be useful in the development of art therapy with the blind, or possibly beyond, and serve towards further studies – of a historical, qualitative or experimental nature: Why has art education pioneer Victor Lowenfeld received so little attention in post-war Central European education and in art therapy at large? Can pre-school blind children benefit from touch-based art-therapy interventions? Can further scrutiny of specific developmental stages in blind children's artwork contribute to a specific curriculum for blind children's art education and to the training needs of their art teachers and art therapists? How can art therapy enter the debate about the possible link between autism and congenital blindness as laid out by Hobson (1993, 2002, 2005), Hobson et al. (1997, 2003) and Pring (2005). It may be intrinsic to the culture of inquiry that a research journey makes us return with more questions than we had when we originally set out.

Notes

1   The entirety of this investigation, especially the case narratives of long-term art therapy, exceeds the scope of this paper and the reader is referred to other sources (Herrmann 2006, 2009, 2010, 2011a, 2011b).

Bibliography

Adelson, E. & Fraiberg, S. (1973), 'Self-representation in language and play: observations of blind children', The Psychoanalytic Quarterly, 42: 539–62.

Adelson, E. & Fraiberg, S. (1974), 'Gross motor development in infants blind from birth', Child Development, 45: 114–26.

Adelson, E. & Fraiberg, S. (1976), 'Sensory deficit and motor development in infants blind from birth', in Z.S. Jastrzembska (ed.) The Effects of Blindness and Other Impairments on Early Development, New York: American Foundation for the Blind.

Burlingham, D. (1961), 'Some notes on the development of the blind', The Psychoanalytic Study of the Child, 16: 121–145

Burlingham, D. (1979), 'To be blind in a sighted world', The Psychoanalytic Study of the Child, 34: 5–30.

Butterworth, G. (1998), 'What is special about pointing in babies?', in F. Simion & G. Butterworth (eds.) The development of Sensory, Motor and Cognitive Capacities in Early Infancy: From Perception to Cognition, Hove: Psychology.

Butterworth, G. & Cochran, E. (1980), 'Towards a mechanism of joint visual attention in human infancy', International Journal of Behavioural Development, 3: 253–72.

Butterworth, G. & Jarrett, N. (1991), 'What minds have in common is space: spatial mechanisms for perspective taking in infancy', British Journal of Developmental Psychology, 9: 55–72.

Creswell, J. (2007), Qualitative Inquiry and Research Design, London: Sage.

Creswell, J. (2009), Research Design. Qualitative, Quantitative, and Mixed Methods Approaches, London: Sage.

Curson, A. (1979), 'The blind nursery school child', The Psychoanalytic Study of the Child, 34: 51–83.

Dalley, T., Rifkind, G. & Terry, K. (1993), Three Voices in Art Therapy. Image, Client, Therapist, London: Routledge.

Damarell, B. (1999), 'Just forging, or seeking love and approval?', Inscape, 4 (2): 44–50.

Damarell, B. (2011), 'Shaping Thoughts: An Investigation into the Cognitive Significance of Image-Making for People with Learning Disabilities', in Gilroy, A. (ed.) Art Therapy Research in Practice, Berne: Peter Lang.

D'Entremont, B., Hains, S. & Muir, D. (1997), 'A demonstration of gaze-following in 3-to-6-months-olds', *Infant Behaviour and Development*, 20: 569–72.

Dryden, W. & Yankura, J. (1992), *Daring to Be Myself*, Buckingham: Open University.

Edwards, D. (1999), 'The role of the case study in art therapy research', *Inscape*, 4 (1): 2–9.

Ezzy, D. (2002), *Qualitative Analysis. Practice and Innovation*, London: Routledge.

Fogel, A. (1997), 'Seeing and Being Seen', in V. Lewis & G. M. Collis (1997) (eds.), *Blindness and Psychological Development in Young Children*, Leicester: BPS.

Fox, M., Martin, P. & Green, G. (2007), *Doing Practitioner Research*, London: Sage.

Fraiberg, S. (1968), 'Parallel and divergent patterns in blind and sighted infants', *The Psychoanalytic Study of the Child*, 23: 264–300.

Fraiberg, S. (1977), *Insights from the Blind*, New York: Basic.

Fraiberg, S. (1979), 'Blind infants and their mothers: an examination of the sign system, in M, Bullowa' (ed.), *Before Speech. The Beginning of interpersonal communication*, Cambridge: Cambridge University.

Fraiberg, S. & Freedman, D. A. (1964), 'Studies in the Ego Development of the Congenitally Blind Child', *The Psychoanalytic Study of the Child*, 19: 113–69.

Gilroy, A. (1992), 'Research in Art Therapy', in D. Waller & A. Gilroy (eds.), *Art Therapy: A Handbook*, Buckingham and Philadelphia: Open University.

Gilroy, A. (2006), *Art Therapy, Research and Evidence-based Practice*, London: Sage.

Hayhoe, S. (2005), 'An Examination of Social and Cultural Factors Affecting Art education in English Schools for the Blind', unpublished doctoral thesis, Birmingham University.

Hayhoe, S. (2008), *God, Money and Politics. English Attitudes to Blindness and Touch from the Enlightenment to Integration*, Charlotte, NC: IAP.

Henley, D. (1991), 'Facilitating the development of object relations through the use of clay in art therapy', *The American Journal of Art Therapy*, 29: 69–76.

Henley, D. (1992), *Exceptional Children. Exceptional Art: Teaching Art to Special Needs*, Worcester, MA: Davis.

Herrmann, U. (1995), 'A Trojan horse of clay: Art therapy in a residential school for the blind', *The Arts in Psychotherapy*, 22 (3): 229–34.

Herrmann, U. (1997), 'A Tangible Reflection. The meaning of sculpture for body image development in art psychotherapy with a congenitally blind client', unpublished Master Thesis, Goldsmiths, University of London.

Herrmann, U. (2001), 'Mein eigenes Haus. Kunsttherapie als Psychotherapie für Kinder und Jugendliche mit NCL', in NCL, *Zur Lebenssituation von blinden Kindern und Heranwachsenden mit einer unheilbaren Abbauerkrankung: Beiträge aus Pädagogik, Therapie und Medizin*, Hanover: Landesbildungszentrum für Blinde/VZFB.

Herrmann, U. (2006), 'Blick und blindheit in der kunsttherapie', *Kunst & Therapie*, 1: 42–54.

Herrmann, U. (2007), 'Does the Self Need an Image? Art Psychotherapy and congenital blindness', Paper given at *In Touch with Art* conference, Victoria & Albert Museum, November 2007.

Herrmann, U. (2009), 'Der Blick der tastenden Hand', in VBS (eds.) *Teilhabe Gestalten*, Würzburg: Edition Bentheim.

Herrmann, U. (2010), 'Braucht das Selbst ein Bild?', in M. Wendlandt-Baumeister, R. Bolle and P. Sinapius (eds.), *Wissenschaftliche Grundlagen der Kunsttherapie*, Berne: Peter Lang.

Herrmann, U. (2011a), ' Tangible Reflection: A single case study investigating body image development in art psychotherapy with a congenitally blind client', in A. Gilroy (ed.) *Art Therapy Research in Practice*, Berne: Peter Lang.

Herrmann, U. (2011b), 'Art Therapy and Congenital Blindness: Investigating the Gaze', unpublished PhD Thesis, Goldsmiths, University of London.

Hobson, R. P. (1993), 'Through Feeling and Sight to Self and Symbol', in U. Neisser (ed.) *The Perceived Self*, Cambridge: Cambridge University.

Hobson, R.P. (2002), *The Cradle of Thought. Exploring the Origins of Thinking*, London: Pan Macmillan.

Hobson, R.P. (2005), 'Beyond Modularity and Innateness: sensory experience, social interaction and symbolic development in children with autism and blindness', in L. Pring (ed.) *Autism and Blindness. Research and Reflections*, London: Whurr.

Hobson, R.P. & Bishop, M. (2003), 'The pathogenis of autism: insights from congenital blindness', *Philosophical Transactions of the Royal Society Biological Sciences* 358, 335–44. Available Online at: www.ncbi.nlm.nih.gov/pmc/articles/PMC1693122/pdf/12639331.pdf (accessed 27 August 2010).

Hobson, R.P., Brown, R., Minter, M. & Lee, A. (1997), 'Autism revisited: the case of congenital blindness', in V. Lewis & G. M. Collis (eds.) *Blindness and Psychological Development in Young Children*. Leister: BPS.

Hockney, D. (2001), *Secret Knowledge. Rediscovering the Lost Techniques of the Old Masters*, London: Thames and Hudson.

Isserow, J. (2008), 'Looking together: joint attention in art therapy', *International Journal of Art Therapy: Inscape*, 13 (1): 34–42.

Isserow, J. (2013), 'Between water and words: reflective self-awareness and symbol formation in art therapy', *International Journal of Art Therapy: Inscape*, 18 (3): 122–31.

Klein, G. S. (1962), 'Blindness and isolation', *The Psychoanalytic Study of the Child*, 17: 82–93.

Kramer, E. (1971) *Art as therapy with children*, New York: Schocken Books.

Kramer, E. (1979) *Childhood and Art Therapy*, New York: Schocken Books.

Kramer, E. (1986), 'The art therapist's third hand: reflections on art, art therapy and society at large', *The American Journal of Art Therapy*, 24 (2): 71–86

Kramer, E. & Gerity, L. A. (eds.) (2000) *Art as Therapy. Collected Papers*, London: Jessica Kingsley.

Landau, B. (1997), Language and Experience in Blind Children: retrospective and prospective, in V. Lewis & G.M. Collis (eds.) *Blindness and psychologic.al development in young children*, Leicester: BPS.

Landau, B. & Gleitman, L.R. (1985), *Language and Experience: Evidence from the blind Child*, Cambridge, MA: Harvard University..

Lowenfeld, V. & Brittain, M. (1957), *Creative and Mental Growth* (5th edn.), New York: Macmillan.

McClelland, S. (1993), The Art of Science with Clients, in H. Payne (ed.) *One River, Many Currents, Handbook of Inquiry in the Arts Therapies*, London: Jessica Kingsley.

McLeod, J. (1994), *Doing Counselling Research*, London: Sage.

McLeod, J. (2001), *Qualitative Research in Counselling and Psychotherapy*, London: Sage

McLeod, J. (2010), *Case Study Research in Counselling and Psychotherapy*, London: Sage.

Mearns, D. & Thorne, B. (1988), *Person-Centred Counselling in Action*, London: Sage.

Michael, J.A (1981), 'Viktor Lowenfeld: Pioneer in Art Education Therapy', *Studies in Art Education*, 22 (2): 7–19.

Michael, J.A (1982), *The Lowenfeld Lectures. Viktor Lowenfeld on Art, Education and Therapy*, Pennsylvania and London: Pennsylvania University.

Olalquiaga, C. (2008), 'Dead Stock: The researcher as collector of failed goods', in M. A. Holly & M. Smith (eds.) *What is Research in the Visual Arts?* New Haven and London: Sterling and Francine Clark Art Institute/Yale University.

Preisler, G. (1997), Social and emotional development of blind children: a longitudinal study, in V. Lewis & G. M. Collis (1997) (eds.) *Blindness and Psychological Development in Young Children*, Leicester: BPS.

Pring, L. (2005), *Autism and Blindness. Research and Reflections*, London: Whurr.

Rehavia-Hanauer, D. (2003), 'Identifying conflicts of anorexia nervosa as manifested in the art therapy process', *The Arts in Psychotherapy*, 30: 137–49.

Rubin, J. (1976), 'The exploration of a "tactile aesthetic"', *New Outlook for the Blind*, 70: 369–75.

Rubin, J. (1978), *Child Art Therapy*, New York: Van Nostrand Reinhold.

Sandler, A. M. (1965), 'Aspects of Passivity and Ego Development in the Blind Infant', *The Psychoanalytic Study of the Child*, 18: 343–60.

Sandler, A. M. & Wills, D. M. (1963), 'Preliminary Notes on Play and Mastery in the Blind Child', *Journal of Child Psychotherapy*, 1 (3): 7–19.

Saunders, R. J. (1960), 'The contributions of Viktor Lowenfeld to art education, Part I: Early influences on his thought', *Studies in Art Education*, 22 (1): 6–15.

Saunders, R. J. (2001), 'Lowenfeld at Penn State: A Remembrance', in S. Corwin (ed.) *Exploring the Legends: Guideposts to the Future*, Reston, VA: NAEA.

Schaverien, J. (1992), *The Revealing Image. Analytical Art Psychotherapy in Theory and Practice*, London: Routledge.

Schaverien, J. (1993), 'The Retrospective Review of Pictures, Data for Research in Art Therapy', in Helen Payne (ed.) *One River, Many Currents. Handbook of Inquiry in the Arts Therapies*, London: Jessica Kingsley.

Schaverien, J. (1995), 'Researching the Esoteric' in A. Gilroy & C. Lee (eds.), *Art and Music Therapy and Research*, London: Routledge.

Sullivan, G. (2010), *Art Practice as Research. Inquiry in Visual Arts*, London: Sage.

Ulman, E. (1987), 'Therapeutic art education by Viktor L. Lowenfeld', *The American Journal of Art Therapy*, 25 (May): 111–46.

Wills, D. M. (1965), 'Some observations on blind nursery school children's understanding of their world', *The Psychoanalytic Study of the Child*, 20: 344–64.

Wills, D. M. (1970), 'Vulnerable periods in the early development of blind children', *The Psychoanalytic Study of the Child*, 25: 461–80.

Wilson, S. (1994), 'On seeing and not seeing', *Journal of Child Psychotherapy*, 20 (2): 165–84.

Wood, M. (2002), 'Researching art therapy practice with people suffering from AIDS-related dementia', *The Arts in Psychotherapy*, 29: 207–19.

Yalom I. & Elkin, G. (1974), *Every Day Gets a Little Closer: A Twice-Told Therapy*, New York: Basic.

Yin, R.K. (2009), *Case Study Research: Design and Methods*, London: Sage.

Chapter 4

Dance movement therapy training

The challenges of interculturality and cross-cultural communication within a diverse student group-analytic large group

Heidrun Panhofer, Peter Zelaskowski and Iris Bräuninger

Introduction

Our masters and postgraduate diploma in dance movement therapy (DMT) at the Autonomous University of Barcelona (UAB)[1] have been running since October 2003 within the complex cultural and political bilingual setting of Catalonia in Spain. Throughout, our student and teacher bodies have been made up of more than twenty different nationalities from Europe (37 per cent: Catalonia; 26 per cent: rest of Spain; 13 per cent: other European countries), South and North America (22 per cent: Mexico, the largest group), Africa and Asia (2 per cent).[2] This tendency towards internationalization is still rising, alongside an increased mobility of students, academics and knowledge, not only at our university, but worldwide (Organization for Economic Cooperation and Development (OECD) 2007; Uvalie-Trumbie, Daniel & West 2007). Some of our students over the past years have been commuting regularly from not only different parts of Spain, but also from Portugal, Switzerland, Germany, France, Ireland, Greece and even Russia. Others leave their home countries behind to come and live in Barcelona, causing the local Catalan students to be a clear minority.

Among the different experiential sessions, which constitute the core of the training, students of the first and second academic years of the course meet on a monthly basis in a large verbal group, conducted along group-analytic lines by an experienced group analyst, within which they are free to discuss any issues of concern to them. The following chapter presents the preliminary findings from a study carried out on this large group, which involved asking all student participants to give a free, written description of the same single session.[3] Using phenomenographic-research methodology (Larsson & Holmström 2007; Marton 1981, 1986), the collected narratives were scrutinized in the light of interculturality.[4]

Interculturality

> The COE, in a project promoting interculturalism in cities, stressed the need for each distinct culture to survive and flourish while defending the right of all cultures to contribute to the cultural landscape of the society in which they are present. The COE thus proposes the development of cultural sensitivity, encouraging intercultural interaction and mixing as an essential aspect of a society: Interculturality derives from the understanding that cultures thrive only in contact with other cultures, not in isolation. It seeks to reinforce intercultural interaction as a means of building trust and reinforcing the fabric of the community.
>
> (Intercultural City 2014, 28 October)

In the light of COE definitions, we would describe our intended approach as intercultural, aiming to include a sociocultural dimension in our training.

> Without first critically examining subtle forms of racial, ethnic, or cultural bias that exist in DMT education and practice, there is a danger of foreclosing communication among socioculturally diverse students and educators, between therapists and clients, and among community participants and facilitators of community-based healing arts events.
>
> (Chang 2009: 300)

The combination within our training of experiential groups, a broad range of supervision and theory classes, as well as the more informal spaces typical of the block-training model, provides multiple spaces within which intercultural exchange can occur. This study deals with one particular experiential space, the large group.

Intercultural communication and sub-grouping: the context of the large group

According to Agazarian's system-centred approach to groups (1987), the underlying dynamic common to the maturation of all human systems, as small as a cell and as large as a society, is the functional discrimination and integration of differences, from the simple to the complex. This model provides a useful framework for describing and making sense of the processes involved in intercultural exchange. Applying Agazarian's model to the context of our training, each cultural group can be thought of as a sub-group of the larger group-as-a-whole and it is through the ongoing process of sub-group interaction that groups engage with their differences and, as a consequence, develop.

> Functional sub-grouping is designed to influence the way that systems function, and it puts into practice the assumption that all living human

systems survive, develop, and transform through the process of discriminating and integrating differences.

(Agazarian 1987)

Within this systems-centred model it is the sub-group, not the individual member, which is the basic unit of the group. For Agazarian (1999), sub-groups serve a clear function, which is to keep the group stable by 'containing' conflicting differences in the group while the group-as-a-whole learns how to integrate them. Sub-group development limits the potential for a more primitive fragmentation that might contribute to the destructive development of an anti-group process (Nitsun 1996). In this sense, in a diverse multicultural training it is the quality of the intercultural communication occurring between the various cultural sub-groups that is the cornerstone of the development and growth of the individuals, as well as of the large group (in the case of this study) and the training as a whole.

Large groups and culture

Large- and median-group theory has been an area of ever-expanding significance and complexity within the field of group-analytic psychotherapy since the pioneering early advocates of large-group theory and practice, Kreeger (1975), De Mare (1972, 1985) and De Mare, Piper & Thompson (1991), who began to focus our attention clearly on the issues of society, culture and citizenship in groups larger than the optimum small group of about eight people. In the large group, the family in which we grew-up is not the core concern. The transference of familial and primitive early patterns of relating is a concept belonging to therapy in small groups. The wider cultural and social context of the individual and the family is more likely activated in the large group. For De Mare (1985) the large group links psychology to sociology. Context (Hopper 1985), in the broadest cultural, social and political sense, is now the fundamental problem and is no longer excluded (De Mare 1985), as it has historically been in psychoanalytic theory. Instead of transference, De Mare *et al.*(1991) speaks of transpositions from previous cultural contexts, which is to say we carry our culture into the large group in the form of macrocultural assumptions, which become transformed in the miniculture of the large group through a process of dialogue. While, for De Mare, it is only in large and median groups that questions of culture can be properly addressed, Weinberg (2003) talks of all group sessions (small, median or large, therapeutic or experiential) as intercultural encounters. Culture grows out of groups; it fills the existential void between the self and others and protects us from primitive anxieties. For Dalal (2001), in his analysis of a radical group-analytic model, there is no self that is separate from culture – even the id itself is acculturated and subject to power, class and racial divisions from the start of life.

While the use of experiential groups in therapist training has significant support in the literature, (e.g. Hutten 1996; Panhofer, García & Zelaskowski 2014; Payne 1999, 2010) there has been much less written about large groups in a training context. A significant exception is Jones and Skaife (2009a & 2009b), writing about a large group within art-therapy training. They stress the potential for institutional and political learning as well as the importance of art in its social and political context.

Culture, context and language

A more recent development in group analysis (Hopper & Weinberg 2011) has seen the emergence of a body of theory around a concept used by Foulkes (1950), the social unconscious, a complex concept with both orthodox and radical forms (Dalal 2001), which is at the heart of the group-analytic project. Among other things, it asks us to pay close attention to the social, cultural and political context in which experience occurs. In other words, what does it mean that this group session took place here in this university, in this city, in this culture? Similarly, Dosamantes (1992), drawing on psychoanalytic theories of individuation and separation, outlines the different stages of group development within a DMT setting, describing how the patterns generated by the body in action reflect the emotional inner life of the person within a particular social context.

In order to provide some sense of the cultural context for the particular group experience in this study, we would like to mention two significant components of the local social unconscious. First, 'el pacto del olvido', the pact of forgetting (Tremlett 2006: 71), a collective unwritten agreement among the Spanish population that bolstered the 1978 Spanish Constitution, considered to be the key in the post-Franco transition to democracy, a determination to leave the past behind and bury historical conflicts and tensions in order to fulfil the democratic objectives enshrined in the constitution. In this sense, a tendency to avoid is as much about leaving out cultural and political issues, in order to leave the past behind, as it is about moving on. The second component is language. Whether it be the second language acquisitional issues of those for whom Castilian Spanish is their second or third language, or the interlinguistic issues brought about by the variety of Castilian Spanish users – mother tongue Spanish, Mexican, Argentinian, etc. and all other national variations. This diversity is equally present within the student group as it is within the staff group. In addition, some Catalan students may struggle to switch from the language of their heart when they drive the couple of kilometres it takes to get to their university in the Catalan capital and attend the DMT course. Linguistic immersion in Catalan is both a policy of the Catalan state and a guiding principle of Catalan culture (Badia i Pujol 2010). Furthermore, Portuguese students mix their mother tongue with the closely connected *Castilian*. Finally, the technical – often English – jargon of psychology, psychotherapy and DMT is regularly translated into a Spanish form, thus helping to construct a new sociolinguistic reality among the students of the course.

Culture, as a learned and shared system of meaning and understanding, is primarily communicated through the means of natural language: 'These meanings and understandings are not just representations about what is in the world; they are also directive, evocative and reality constructing in character' (D'Andrade's 1990: 65).

Wittgenstein (1953) pointed out the inseparability of language and context, underlining the social event that happens between the users of a language. He compares language with an old town that grows over time, with its lanes and squares, new and old buildings from different *époques*, surrounded by different suburbs with their straight and linear streets (Wittgenstein 1953). The meaning of language to him is a complicated phenomenon that is woven into the fabric of our lives, just like the life of our training and the intercultural exchange it provides at all times.

Phenomenography as a research methodology

The methodological framework used, which is broadly speaking phenomenographic, stems from a basic original objective, which was to describe a single session of an experiential group from the point of view of all of its participants (Larsson & Holmström 2007). The phenomenographic-research method seemed particularly appropriate. First, it is grounded in the exploration of how specific phenomena are experienced by those taking part. Second, it has the basic objective of elucidating and categorizing variation in ways of experiencing the same phenomenon. Originally developed by Marton (1981), the phenomenographic method explores the similarities and differences in ways of experiencing learning. Understanding variations in how learning is experienced by students can '. . . facilitate educators to improve students' learning outcomes, and provide a foundation for developing more appropriate curricula or instructional approaches' (Hung-Ming Lin 2011: 2).

According to Marton, the aim of phenomenography is '. . . to find and systematize forms of thought in terms of which people interpret aspects of reality – aspects which are socially significant and which are at least supposed to be shared by the members of a particular kind of society' (1981: 180).

With this research we were interested in bringing together these different aspects of reality, allowing the different members of the group from their different cultures to share their part of the experience of a large verbal group.

Procedures

The original research goal was to generate a multi-subjective description of a single learning experience. In order to make sense of the subjective experiences of our students, a five-step model was developed.

Table 4.1 shows the applied five-step procedures.

Table 4.1 Flow chart to illustrate the pathway through the research process

Step 1 Data collection	Step 2 Data collection	Step 3 Data analysis	Step 4 Data analysis	Step 5 Data Findings
Large group	Participants in large group write narratives	Researcher 1 scrutinized the texts and identified some initial categories	Researcher 2 searches for intercultural themes: where did writers make reference to their own belonging to a specific sub-group, where did they identify other groups, refer to the group as a whole etc.? Researcher 1 searches for intercultural themes: where did writers make reference to their own belonging to a specific sub-group, where did they identify other groups, refer to the group as a whole etc.?	Comparison of the findings of co-researcher 1 and 2, interpretation of the findings

Step 1: Students participated in a one-hour group-analytic large-group session, the ninth in a series of ten sessions within one academic year of the DMT training.

Step 2: The forty-six participants of the group were asked to give a free written description of the session immediately afterwards, thus reducing the possibilities of interpersonal contamination of subjective descriptions and hopefully maximizing the variety and individuality of perspective, i.e., facilitating each individual's subjective remembering and describing.

Step 3: Subsequently, two of the authors analysed the material in a way described by Wolcott (1994, 2001). The qualitative data were transformed through categorization. Researcher 1 scrutinized the texts and identified some initial categories.[5]

Step 4: Researchers 1 and 2 looked for: comments relating to national belonging and for emerging intercultural themes; references to belonging to specific sub-groups; comments identifying other groups; and any references to the group-as-a-whole, etc.

Step 5: Subsequently, both researchers' findings were compared.

The following interpretation of the key factors and patterns according to Wolcott (2001: 33) was not

> derived from rigorous, agreed-upon, carefully specified procedures, but from our efforts at sense making, a human activity that included intuition, past experience, emotion – personal attributes of human researchers that can be argued endlessly but neither proved nor disproved to the satisfaction of all.

These qualitative procedures provided us with a means of reflecting on the diversity of the lived experience of our students. Initially, this investigation was not directed at the phenomenon of interculturality as such, but through the use of phenomenographic methods certain variations in the students' ways of addressing cultural themes became apparent (Larsson & Holmström 2007).

Findings

A previous research (Panhofer 2011), comparing written accounts by therapists and patients, shows the incredible divergence between accounts, at times even giving the impression that therapist and client had been in different spaces. Similarly, in this research, the accounts of one single group session were at times very different – varying in length (from 144 words min. to 1100 words max.) – and quality, and ranging from aloof third-person descriptions to very private accounts, including personal reflections, emotions, physical states and images. Given the large number of accounts (thirty five), the researchers who had not been physically present in the session and who analysed the written material were nonetheless able to form a broader, multi-subjective picture of what had happened during the session.

The group as a container

The process of organizing and reporting of the data beyond the purely descriptive account allowed us to identify certain key factors and patterns, as well as the relationships between them. During Step 3 of the procedures, the first common pattern emerged: most of the imagery was concerned with inside and outside, making reference to a container and one's personal position regarding this container, for example 'the setting like a uterus'[6] (Student 29), 'forming part of a species' (Student 33), 'the group as a womb' (Student 24), 'the barrier between me and the group' (Student 1), 'feeling outside' (Student 1), 'wanting to break through my own boundaries' (Student 2), etc.

A common thread described the container as a construct of values set up by the group, in the context of a large verbal group, many times connected with either talking or remaining in silence: 'the session started, as usual, with a silence' (Student 2), 'there was a period of about 20 minutes of silence' (Student 4), 'I think the initial silence took longer than usual' (Student 6), 'the usual silence starts to invade the space and the facial expressions' (Student 1), 'I wanted to say it but breaking the silence is difficult' (Student 8), 'I wanted to ask the group (. . .) but I didn't. I thought that perhaps they did not want to share in such a large group if they were not doing well' (Student 25), 'for a moment I disconnect from the conversation and withdraw into myself' (Student 24), 'the group has taught me on a more practical level – being able to speak, deal with the silence, being able not to speak' (Student 25), 'I think I still have not understood or digested my own silence' (Student 2), etc.

National identity

Only very view comments actually spoke about national identity:

> After a few coughs, a colleague expresses that in her head she has an image of a large beer and refers to her culture, she is English (British)
>
> (Student 26)

> 'The first person intervenes . . . with an extended comment on a personal fantasy about beer, football and her nationality'
>
> (Student 24)

> 'I managed to keep listening and to understand what people were saying even though this is not my language'
>
> (Student 11)

> 'In this moment a Chilean woman responded. She sat right behind me and just by hearing her tone of voice (she had already done it before in this session) I felt a movement in my belly, similar to a boiling kettle. I did not know what would be her 'contribution' and I am putting this into brackets because generally I feel that this girl never contributes anything, she only complicates the flow of things and seeks attention'
>
> (Student 14)

These few comments either pick up statements from other group members (Students 26 and 24) or make reference to one's personal limitations due to a lack of linguistic skills (Student 11). Only in one case is a particular person pointed to in a negative way, adding her nationality as some kind of specific information on her personality (Student 14). However, the student does not extend her negative statement to 'all Chileans', but rather she uses nationality as a means of identifying, instead of naming, a particular person.

Intercultural themes

During Step 4 of the data analysis both researchers highlighted a series of intercultural themes understanding culture as a system of meanings and symbols that is historically transmitted (Geertz 1973). The researchers looked at themes of shared identity and common meanings and selected text whenever students made reference to their belonging to a specific sub-group, where they identified other groups or referred to the group-as-a-whole. Both researchers coincided with their chosen material in 71 per cent of the selected writings, showing some differences mainly in themes around the group facilitator (one researcher included these as belonging to 'intercultural themes' whereas the other did not). Here are a series of examples of material chosen by both researchers:

> I connect to the notion that the group needs to re-connect itself every single time it meets because it only exists, at least in my experience, in this space and time physically and symbolically.
>
> (Student 19)

> As with every weekend when it is time to attend this class I thought: no! Again, I have to meet with these people in this space, this narrow place, but perhaps what I feared most was not the people, nor the experience. Given that when you feel well and you speak well this place and these people can turn into something entertaining.
>
> (Student 9)

> Today the group spoke about individuality and collectivism. The group that exists and is part of us, no matter if we are present or how we experience the group. The group leaves a trace of every individual, the individual forms part of the group, even if absent.
>
> (Student 32)

> They ask her about her attachment to the large group and she says she has no particular fondness for it. My sensation is similar, I get the experience but there are peers with whom I have not yet formed an attachment.
>
> (Student 3)

Sub-group identity

Sub-groups were often defined in terms of first and second year students: 'the girls in the back from the first year' (Student 15), 'I think that the roles of the first and second year have been very present during the entire year' (Student 12), 'my sensation of the group is that the division between first and second year had diluted a bit' (Student 31), or

> I wanted to express my thoughts concerning the continuity of the group, directing myself to those from the first year, but I didn't, in order not to enter into a first-and-second-year-dichotomy.
>
> (Student 34)

> Several people knock with the back of their fists on the chair and it is mentioned that this code has been established by the sub-group of first-year students to show that they share the opinion or emotion of somebody.
>
> (Student 24)

Most importantly, a common theme of those who spoke and those who did not occurred, describing different sub-cultures of the large verbal group:

> He [*the facilitator, note of the authors*] made reference to a sub-group that has been created, situated where I found myself sitting today. He said he had been aware of this already for a few sessions and exactly today, when I find myself in this very place, he names it.
>
> (Student 7)

> I became nervous and felt the tension generated in the group. At the beginning of the course I used to sit there intending to hide because I did not want to participate; I feel that today I am re-living this sensation and I am happy to see that it has gone and I now feel part of this group.
>
> (Student 10)

> Just like the sub-group that hides within the group through its silence.
>
> (Student 3)

> These people who do not speak, this special ghetto or slum, are they included among the people? Or are we one divided country where only those who speak are listened to?
>
> (Student 22)

> I thought: Why is he putting pressure? Why discriminate? Why make differences and name people who do not speak as a 'suburb'? Is this not dividing and separating? Are we not supposed to be one group with a large range of personalities, interests and differences? I felt that suddenly we belonged to a 'type' of group where my free choice to be as I am was not respected, and that we had to enter pre-designed dynamics.
>
> (Student 18)

> X (who was in this suburb) asks Peter directly (*the facilitator, note of the authors*) if he too actually hides. I sense that she does this, moved by the threat to her suburb.
>
> (Student 17)

> When the person responsible for the 'slum of silence' spoke, it was like saying that the words were so important that they have power for every person.
>
> (Student 29)

A central and constant theme within the large group of speaking or remaining in silence, as well as the importance of the spoken word, emerged.

Shared norms

Sometimes students referred to an established set of values and the sense of being judged according to the group's norms:

> I identify a lot with the ideas of some regarding the complexity of interaction in the large group, it is something that provokes physical and psychical effects in me. When I think about the impossibility of the other understanding my subjectivity, I get anxious and isolate myself. In fact, this is one of my apprehensions about the large group and it is this idea, which blocks me when it comes to participating in the group dialogue.
>
> (Student 19)

> I only added to what I had said, that it was part of my vision, a phrase I am lately using more and more frequently and firmly in order to defend myself and my form of existence. Why do we have to defend ourselves? Why do I have the feeling and the image that today's session was like a tribunal, a judgement where everybody feels the necessity to defend themselves and to judge others?
>
> (Student 23)

The emerging set of values and the sense of being judged may be linked to the group culture, but may also address the complexity of working experientially within an academic context (see Panhofer *et al.* 2014; Payne 1999, 2010) where free expression of feelings may collide with traditional academic values, which overvalue the quantifiable and objective measure at the expense of the qualitative and subjective.

Discussion

The above vignettes are suggestive of a tendency for students to avoid referencing themes indicative of cultural diversity (whether national, linguistic or otherwise) and by extension sidestepping any concomitant cultural tensions. This could also, however, be connected to language and setting. Despite the culture of linguistic immersion predominant in Catalan institutional life, the vehicular language of the course is Spanish, *Castellano* as referred to in Spain, from *Castilia*, the very heart of Spain. In our case, this means an intercultural encounter between a variety of forms of Spanish/Castilian, involving: Spanish students from many different parts of Spain; Latin Americans from Central and South America; and Catalan students who speak mainly Catalan as their mother tongue and Spanish as a second language. But, the group also contains international students from a range of other places who are using Spanish as their second or third language, finding themselves sometimes in the paradoxical situation of still having to learn a language in order to communicate and to communicate in order to learn (Roberts 2014).

The common Spanish language in our course facilitates cultural interaction and promotes assimilation and adaptation. The writings allowed us to have a trace of the students' multi-subjective description of a single learning experience. With our training being a masters and postgraduate degree in DMT, there are other learning spaces where experience depends much less on verbal communication. A series of lectures and experiential classes, connected to the dynamics of DMT or movement observation and analysis, focus solely on embodied experience and non-verbal communication. In this study, however, we do not look at intercultural themes from a purely non-verbal viewpoint, as provided by Chang (2006, 2009), Dokter (1998), Moore and Yamamoto (2011), Pallaro (1997), Pylvänäinen (2008) and Stanton-Jones (1992).

The tendency to not mention or sublimate intercultural themes, we suggest, may also be connected with the social unconscious of the majority local culture, as well as to 'the need to fit in' and to avoid attracting attention by remaining within the confines of academic conformism. One student mentioned:

> The response of the group shows me that nobody wants to emphasize the differences in order to 'keep the party in peace', without complications, tensions, crisis. Once again I feel that people tend to avoid crisis.
>
> (Student 28)

Another student emphasizes even more the necessity to adapt:

> As if they do not participate in the group because they are not interested in it, or because they don't want to show themselves. I don't like to show myself either but I follow the instructions of the group. I try to adapt. The facilitator has drawn attention to the area in the group as being like a cultural suburb. What came to my mind was the culture of the group this year of keeping the door open and disorganizing the space.
>
> (Student 27)

The image of 'embracing the difference within the group' emerges:

> We said that the same happens here, we are all very different. One peer refers to the fact that there are many differences in the group, but they have not emerged. Another colleague says that perhaps it would be better to 'embrace our differences'.
>
> (Student 26)

This image of embracing differences is also picked up and referenced by others (Students 17, 26, 34) and seems to express a desire to co-exist peacefully, respecting the differences among the group members.

Instead of an open intercultural confrontation, cross-cultural communication becomes sublimated and expressed through other more immediate and less culturally and politically sensitive sub-groups, such as generational identities (first- and second-year groups), professional identities (dancers/movers or psychologists, contemporary or classical trained dancers, etc.), those who speak in the group and those who do not, etc., promoting withdrawal into cultural and not national sub-groupings.

> In the end I sat next to my friends who are my group of reference and who give me confidence, security and even identity as a member of the large group.
>
> (Student 4)

> When I saw this in a colleague who formed part of my sub-group I felt as if it had been me who had been talking.
>
> (Student 9)

> For me it is hard to speak in groups . . . and this is why it is easier to cut myself from the group and have my own sub-group so I don't have to notice what is going on. That way I don't have to face the struggle if I should or should not speak. At least this way I don't have to feel this dilemma, not to feel the physical struggle of constriction, tension and control.
>
> (Student 15)

By identifying with specific sub-groups some of the potential benefits of intercultural (as distinct from multicultural) communication are eroded.

Chang (2006, 2009) states that cultural consciousness in DMT education and training is generally not sufficiently addressed. She demands a deeper exploration of one's sociocultural identify in order to be able to work success-fully with clients, colleagues and community members from different back-grounds. We agree with Chang on the importance of addressing and working through one's own cultural identity and exploring one's personal habitus

(Bourdieu 1977) during the course of a DMT training. From our experience, however, we also see that intercultural issues cannot always be addressed in a direct manner but may need to emerge via different themes of sub-grouping. Weinberg (2003) warns how groups can become blocked and stuck in the differentiation phase of development. The effectiveness of groups with people coming from many different cultures is determined by how much its members feel free to discuss their feelings about the group. Only when members of the group feel free to express criticism or caring for each other can the group advance effectively (White 1994).

Qing, Schweisfurth and Daya (2009) confirm the co-existence of belonging and alienation for international students who are exposed to intercultural experiences. Learners initially fear and then appreciate the new ways of learning. In order to survive successfully, students must create a coherent trajectory out of these fragments and contradictions: 'The cross-cultural is not only within the intercultural: it is within themselves' (Qing et al. 2009: 14).

During the particular large group session researched, important themes such as talking or remaining in silence emerged, and sub-cultures relating to who does or who doesn't speak were clearly identified among the group. This has clearly helped many students to identify these intercultural themes within themselves; for example, when one student explained eloquently:

> I am saying good-bye with words because thanks to words I can bring all this into an order, thanks to words I can live in 'slums', knowing that one day I can move to another part of the town, knowing that I won't need to hide in these ghettos any more . . . but I hope the moment will come when I will be able to express myself.
>
> (Student 9)

Developing the capacity of DMT students to express themselves and to communicate verbally is of course an important component of the training, just as it is in academic culture, as well within this group-analytic

Limitations

As our research project is qualitative in nature, our results cannot be generalized. The common Spanish language may at times iron-out or homogenize cultural difference. Undoubtedly, some of the micro- and macro-conditions of discourse present in the writings of the students were lost, too, either during the course of its first translation into Spanish (some international students chose to write in their mother tongue and were asked to translate their writing into Spanish), or during the second translation into English, realized by the authors for this book chapter. Thus a lot of the original linguistic and cultural richness was certainly 'lost in translation' (Hoffman 1989, title) an important characteristic and certainly a limitation of this study.

Conclusions

The examination and analysis of the students' writings have shown clearly that intercultural themes tended to be avoided, i.e., not directly confronted, but were, nonetheless, present having been sublimated and disguised in other forms. We argue that most probably this is an indicator of these issues being either too threatening or considered irrelevant by the students to their core academic and training goals, whether because of the academic setting or the constellation of the training group. Instead, other themes of sub-grouping emerge around criteria connected to the university background, such as generational, professional, verbal and non-verbal, etc. identities. Bearing in mind intercultural issues as we encounter them in our training and within the Catalan reality is certainly vital. However, we also recognize that they can be worked through via other issues of personal and sub-group identity. We suggest that the cross-cultural does not only exist within intercultural exchanges, but is within every individual and can be worked through in any group and individuation process.

Appendix

During the first ten generations (from 2003–2013) the programme hosted a total of 314 total students, 106 from the postgraduate degree and 208 from the Master's programme.

37 per cent from Catalonia (83 students); 26 per cent from the rest of Spain (five from Andalusia, five from Aragon, two from the Balearic Islands, three from the Canary Islands, two from Cantabria, four from Castillia and León, two from Extremadura, three from Galicia, one from La Rioja, nine from Madrid, twelve from the Basque Country and nine from Valencia).

PROCEDENCIA FÍSICA ALUMNOS

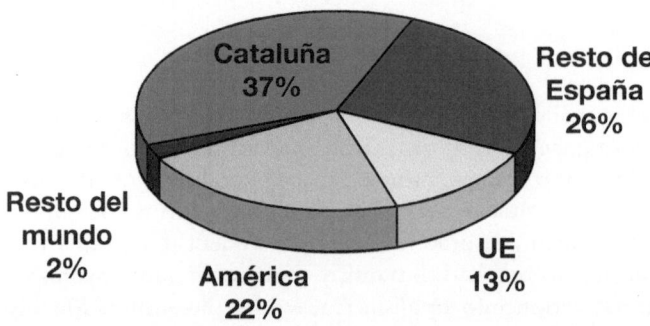

Figure 4.1 The geographical origin of the students

Source: Lleonart 2014: 222

A total of 26 per cent of the students are from other European countries (one student from Andorra, one from the UK, one from Russia, one from Switzerland, one from Germany, two from Greece, two from Holland, two from Ireland, three from Italy, six from France and ten from Portugal), and commute either from their country of origin, or reside in Barcelona for the duration of the course.

A total of 22 per cent of the students come from North and South America (one from Puerto Rico, one from Argentina, one from Cuba, one from the Dominican Republic, one from Ecuador, one from Peru, one from Uruguay, one from the USA, one from Brazil, two from Venezuela, seven from Colombia, eleven from Chile and twenty one from Mexico). 2 per cent of the students have their origin in other countries, with one student from Taiwan and one from Morocco.

Notes

1 The programme is psychodynamically orientated and includes a strong basis combining Laban movement observation and analysis and the Kestenberg Movement Profile.
2 These numbers refer to the first years of the Master's Programme (2003–2013); see Appendix I in Panhofer & Ratés (2014).
3 Informed consent was sought so the material could be analysed and published.
4 Peter Zelaskowski was the group analyst of this particular large group, the two researchers the other authors of the chapter: Researcher 1 Heidrun Panhofer and Researcher 2 Iris Bräuninger
5 Some of those early categories created were subsequently discarded as the research developed and became more focused.
6 All original Spanish writings were translated into English language by the authors of this chapter.

Bibliography

Agazarian, Y. M. (1987), 'Group-as-a-Whole Theory Applied to Scapegoating', unpublished paper supplementary to the workshop on 'Deviance, Scapegoating and Group Development' at the Eastern Group Psychotherapy Conference, New York.

Agazarian, Y. M. (1999), 'Phases of Development in the Systems-Centered Psychotherapy Group', Small Group Research, 30: 82.

Badia i Pujol, J. (2010), 'Gràcies a la immersió lingüística', Revista Òmnium, 15. Available online at: www.omnium.cat/docroot/omnium/includes/news/fitxers/4547/RevistaOmnium15-article-immersio.pdf (accessed 12 November 2014).

Bourdieu, P. (1977), Outline of a Theory of Practice. R. Nice, trans. Cambridge: Cambridge University.

Chang, M. (2006), 'How do Dance/Movement Therapists Bring Awareness of Race, Ethnicity, and Cultural Diversity Into their Practice?', in S. C. Koch & I. Bräuninger (eds.), Advances in Dance/Movement Therapy: Theoretical perspectives and empirical findings (pp. 192–205). Berlin: Logos.

Chang, M. (2009), 'Cultural Consciousness and the Global Context of Dance/ Movement Therapy', in S. Chaiklin, & H. Wengrower (eds.), *The Art and Science of Dance/Movement Therapy: life is dance* (pp. 299–312), New York: Routledge.

COE – Intercultural City: Governance and Policies for Diverse Communities. Available online at: www.coe.int/t/dg4/cultureheritage/culture/Cities/Interculturality_en.pdf (accessed 28 October 2014).

Dalal, F. (2001), 'The Social Unconscious: a post-Foulkesian perspective', *Group Analysis*, 34 (4): 539–55.

D'Andrade, R. (1990), Some Propositions About the Relations Between Culture and Human Cognition, in J. W Stingler, R. A. Shweder, & G. Herdt, (eds.), *Cultural Psychology: essays on comparative human development* (pp. 65–129). New York: Cambridge University.

De Mare, P. (1972), 'Large group psychotherapy: a suggested technique', *Group Analysis*, 5: 106–08.

De Mare, P. (1985), 'Large group perspectives', *Group Analysis*, 18: 78–92.

De Mare, P., Piper, R. & Thompson, S. (1991), *Koinonia: From Hate through Dialogue to Culture in the Larger Group*, London: Karnac.

Dokter, D. (ed.) (1998), *Arts Therapists, Refugees, and Migrants: Reaching across borders*, London: Jessica Kingsley.

Foulkes, S. H. (1950), 'A short survey and orientation with particular reference to Group Analysis', *British Journal of Medical Psychology*, 23: 199–205.

Geertz, C. (1973), *The Interpretation of Cultures*, New York: Basic.

Hoffman, E. (1989), *Lost in Translation: A life in a new language*, London: Random House.

Hopper, E. (1985), 'The Problem of Context in Group Analytic Psychotherapy: A clinical illustration and brief theoretical discussion', in M. Pines (ed.), *Bion and Group Psychotherapy*. London: Routledge.

Hopper, E. & Weinberg, H. (2011), *The Social Unconscious in Persons, Groups and Societies. Volume 1: Mainly Theory*, London: Karnac.

Hung-Ming L. (2011), 'A Phenomenographic Approach for Exploring Conceptions of Learning Marketing among Undergraduate Students', *Business and Economic Research*, 1: 1–12. Available online at: www.macrothink.org/journal/index.php/ber/article/download/829/1602, (28 October 2014).

Hutten, J. M. (1996), 'The use of experiential groups in the training of counsellors and psychotherapists', *Psychodynamic Counselling*, 2: 247–56.

Jones, K. & Skaife, S. (2009a), 'Under the cobblestones, the beach: the politics and possibilities of the art therapy large group', *Psychotherapy and Politics International*, 7: 18–27.

Jones K. & Skaife, S. (2009b), 'The art therapy large group as a teaching method for the institutional and political aspects of professional training', *Learning in Heath Care & Social Care*, 8: 200–09.

Kreeger, L. (ed.) (1975), *The Large Group: Dynamics and Therapy*, London: Constable.

Larsson, J. & Holmström, I. (2007), 'Phenomenographic or phenomenological analysis: does it matter? Examples from a study on anaesthesiologists' work', *International Journal of Qualitative Studies on Health and Well-being*, 2: 55–64.

Lleonart, N. (2014), 'Estadísticas', in H Panhofer (ed.) *Encontrar – Compartir – Aprender. 10° aniversario del master en Danza Movimiento Terapia, Universitat Autònoma de Barcelona*. Bellaterra: UAB Servei de Publicacions.

Marton, F. (1981), 'Phenomenography – describing conceptions of the world around us', *Instructional Science*, 10: 177–200.

Marton, F. (1986), 'Phenomenography: A research approach to investigating different understandings of reality', *Journal of Thought*, 21: 28–49.

Moore, C. L. & Yamamoto, K. (2011), *Beyond Words. Movement Observation and Analysis* (2nd edn), London: Gordon and Breach.

Nitsun, M. (1996), *The Anti-Group*. London: Routledge.

Organization for Economic Cooperation and Development (OECD) (2007). *Globalisation and higher education*. Paris: OECD.

Pallaro, P. (1997), 'Culture, self and body-self: dance/movement therapy with Asian Americans', *The Arts in Psychotherapy*, 24: 227–41

Panhofer, H. (2011), 'Languaged and non-languaged ways of knowing in counselling and psychotherapy', *British Journal of Guidance & Counselling*, 39: 455–70.

Panhofer, H. & Ratés A. (eds.) (2014), *'Encontrar – Compartir – Aprender', Jornadas del 10° aniversario del Máster en Danza Movimiento Terapia*. Barcelona: Universitat Autònoma de Barcelona. Available online at: https://ddd.uab.cat/pub/llibres/2014/117258/enccomapr_a2014.pdf (accessed 28 October 2014).

Panhofer, H., García, M. E., & Zelaskowski, P. (2014), 'The challenge of working with embodied, emotional consciousness in the context of a university-based Dance Movement Therapy training', *The Arts in Psychotherapy*, 41: 115–19.

Payne, H. (1999), 'Personal development groups in the training of counsellors and therapists: a review of the research', *European Journal of Psychotherapy & Counselling*, 2: 55–68.

Payne, H. (2010), 'Personal development groups in post graduate movement psychotherapy training: a study examining the contribution to practice', *The Arts in Psychotherapy*, 37 (3): 202–10.

Pylvänäinen, P. (2008), 'A dance/movement therapy group as a community outreach for intercultural women in Tokyo', *Body, Movement and Dance in Psychotherapy: An International Journal for Theory, Research and Practice*, 3: 31- 44, doi: 10.1080/1743 2970701717767.

Qing, G., Schweisfurth, M. & Daya, C. (2009), 'Learning and growing in a "foreign" context: intercultural experiences of international students', *British Association for International and Comparative Education: iFirst Article*, 1–17.

Roberts, C. (2014), 'Background to the Understanding Project', in K. Bremer & C. Roberts (eds.) *Achieving Understanding: discourse in intercultural encounters* (pp. 1–8), London: Routledge.

Stanton-Jones, K. (1992), *Dance Movement Therapy in Psychiatry*, London: Routledge.

Tremlett, G. (2006), *Ghosts of Spain*, London: Faber and Faber.

Uvalie-Trumbie, S., Daniel, J., & West, P. (2007), 'The role of international online courses in the worldwide provision of education', paper presented at the *European Association of Distance Teaching Universities 20th Anniversary Conference*, September 8–9, Lisbon.

Weinberg, H. (2003), 'The culture of the group and groups from different cultures', *Group Analysis*, 36: 253–68.

White, J. C. (1994), 'The impact of race and ethnicity on transference and counter-transference in combined individual-group therapy', *Group*, 18: 89–99.

Wittgenstein, L. (1953), *Philosophical Investigations*, G.E.M. Anscombe, Trans., New York: Macmillan.

Wolcott, H. (1994), *Transforming Qualitative Data: Description, Analysis, and Interpretation.* London: Sage.

Wolcott, H. (2001), *Writing Up Qualitative Research*, London: Sage.

Chapter 5

Transposing musical cultures in music therapy

Exploring the use of Indonesian gamelan music in western clinical practice

Helen Loth

Introduction

This study was borne out of the experience of the author as a music therapist and as a gamelan player. The gamelan is an ensemble of instruments on which the traditional music of Indonesia is played. Music therapy practice in the UK is grounded in improvisation and live music-making, while also making use of pre-composed and recorded music (British Association for Music Therapy 2012). The range of instruments used generally includes tuned and un-tuned percussion, some orchestral instruments, keyboards and some world percussion instruments (Bunt & Hoskyns 2002; Darnley-Smith & Patey 2003). These are selected to be playable by clients with no musical training. There are no reports of the use of an entire ensemble of non-Western musical instruments in music therapy practice.

While there has been discussion about how Western music therapy practice (and music) is imported to Asian cultures (Futamata 2005; Chong 2009, 2010) there is little research and literature about how Eastern music therapy practice and music can be imported to the West. Moreno (1988) argues that music therapists should learn about a wide range of world-music genres and includes Balinese gamelan as an example of this. However, he makes suggestions for using the basic musical structures of gamelan to play on Orff[1] percussion instruments rather than using the gamelan instruments themselves. Some music therapy training programmes include practical experiences of music from different cultures as a way of broadening the therapists' improvisational resources. As Pavlicevic (1997) points out, music from different cultures contains differences in 'musical energy'. Through becoming familiar with these, music therapists can draw from different musical genres, styles and idioms in their improvisation to 'reflect or evoke something within the client's playing' (Pavlicevic 1997: 37).

A series of discussions in the international online music therapy forum 'Voices' addressed issues arising from musicians from Asian countries, training in Western music therapy courses and returning home to practice. Acknowledging the tendency for music therapists to replicate Western practice,

Futamata (2005), in an article entitled 'Things Asian Music Therapists Should Learn' exhorts Japanese music therapists who have trained in Europe and the US not to ignore the resources they have as Japanese and Asian therapists. These include the music and instruments as well as human relationships, aesthetics and spiritual traditions. Chong (2010) gives the example of how the traditional form of Korean singing, known as 'Sori' was researched for its therapeutic potential (voicing) in music therapy practice in Korea. The discussion emphasizes that Eastern cultures have much to teach Western music therapists and that the understanding and sharing of the therapeutic properties of both Western and Eastern music would benefit all music therapists.

Gamelan music is becoming increasingly well known and played in the UK. Since the first sets of gamelan instruments arrived in in the late 1970s and early 1980s, their number has steadily increased to over a hundred sets. These are mainly being used in universities, schools, orchestral centres and community arts settings. The context of this work is broadly educational. More recently, these instruments are also being used in music groups with children and adults with a range of specific needs, such as those with learning disabilities or mental health problems, the hearing impaired, young offenders and prisoners (Palmer 1991; Ingram 1997; Smith 1997; Hawley 2005; Mendonca 2010). Group sessions range from one-off workshops, intensive week-long projects or weekly classes and are run by gamelan tutors. While most of this work appears to be undertaken in an educational or recreational context, some literature points to the therapeutic benefits of particular pieces of work. These reports suggest that gamelan playing may have potential applications within music therapy practice that could usefully be explored by a music therapist and could offer new knowledge for music therapy theory and practice. This was the focus of the research study.

Summary of research study

The study was designed to investigate in a systematic manner what the therapeutic benefits of gamelan playing could be, and to make suggestions for how these might be used in music therapy clinical practice. It sought to answer the main research question: 'What does the playing of gamelan music have to offer the practice of music therapy?' It consisted of two main parts. The first investigated the current and past use of gamelan with people who have a range of special needs, and considered the therapeutic benefits of this. Literature and research relevant to this subject were reviewed and the practice of gamelan tutors in special-needs gamelan workshops and classes were investigated through a mapping exercise and semi-structured interviews. The findings of the first part were then taken and applied to the practice of music therapy in the second part of the study, through a series of music therapy sessions using gamelan with children with learning disabilities. Finally, a synthesis of all the data was undertaken to answer the main research question, of what the playing of gamelan music has to offer the practice of music therapy. A set of principles for using gamelan in music therapy was developed and suggestions made for clinical applications.

The gamelan

Gamelan is a generic term to describe an ensemble of instruments on which the traditional music of Indonesia is played. An ensemble consists of tuned gongs, (suspended and horizontal), and metallophones, usually made from bronze, wooden xylophones, drums, a two-stringed bowed instrument, a zither-type instrument, bamboo flutes and singers. There are many different types of sets of instruments originating in different parts of Indonesia with different styles of music attached to them; however, they share the same basic instrument types and musical structures. A gamelan ensemble can consist of between about five and twenty-five instruments and players. The instruments are tuned to four-, five- or seven-tone scales, and are frequently elaborately carved and painted, making them very striking to look at. The two principle traditions of gamelan are found in Java and Bali, respectively, two of the most populated Indonesian islands. The research study focused on these, which are the most commonly known of, and found, in the UK and the West. Most gamelan music shares a basic structure. This comprises the core melody (or series of melodies), the gongs marking subdivisions of the melody, (scaffolding), the elaborations of the core melody, and the drumming patterns. Pieces have differing musical forms, modes and tunings. Given the core melody or musical outline of a piece, a musician will be able to construct other parts according to known conventions of the types of pieces and roles of instruments.

Literature review

A review of ethnomusicology literature revealed several aspects of the music and its place in society that have relevance to the research questions. Gamelan

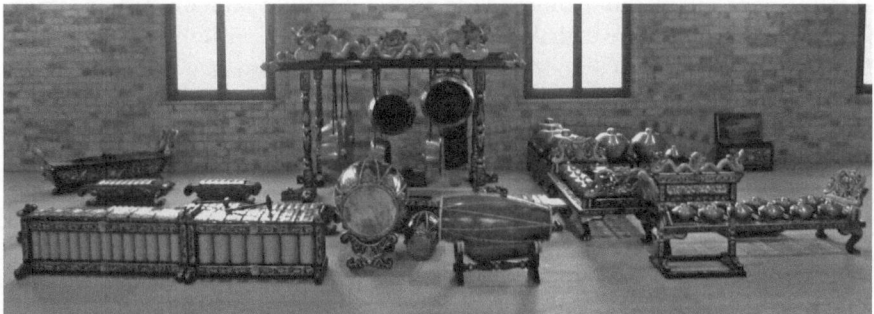

Figure 5.1 A Javanese gamelan set

music is linked to many aspects of life and religion in Indonesia. It is an essential accompaniment to dance, various forms of theatre such as dance-drama, and shadow-puppet plays (wayang kulit), which are widely practised arts. The range of settings and purposes of gamelan playing in Java include 'entertainment, ritual, education, meditation or commemoration of special events' (Brinner 2008: 4). In Bali, the gamelan is an essential part of village life and the life of the temple, of which every village has at least three (Gold 2005). It is played at the many festivals and ceremonies occurring in the temples throughout the year. In addition, gamelan in Bali is also played at many secular events, for performance to dignitaries and in gamelan competitions and festivals.

In addition to the court gamelan and music schools and academies in Java, there are many amateur groups. Javanese children learn some simple gamelan in school, and some continue to play in adulthood in these groups. Many businesses and workplaces have their own gamelan group, which mainly serves a social function; this is somewhere to meet and talk together, as well as play some music, generally led by a professional musician (Brinner 2008). An important feature of social gamelan playing in Java is that people from all sections of society can mix and the traditional hierarchies are broken down.

Reflections in the music of Indonesian society

Many Western and Indonesian writers have pointed out the links between the communal aspects of Indonesian society and gamelan music: 'Gamelan music in Java and Bali provides a model of traditional society in sonic form' (Spiller 2008: 105). Central to Indonesian society is the importance of the community, and the value given to collectiveness over individuality. Brinner (1995) describes how the ensemble nature of the music reflects the values and working of society, describing the basic Javanese social concepts that can be applied to the music as 'rukun', (meaning compatibility or cooperation) and 'gotong royong' (meaning mutual cooperation, working together in harmony)' (Brinner 1995: 292). These values apply to many areas of life, and are integral to the successful playing of the music. In addition, Brinner links the Javanese behavioural ideal of refinement and a calm manner to the music: 'Ideally a Javanese person strives to maintain equilibrium verbally, physically, and emotionally' (Brinner 1995: 293). This is an ideal in a good Javanese musical performance too.

Describing Balinese gamelan, Gold (2005) links cultural values and the music explicitly: 'Balinese music is primarily an ensemble tradition, reflecting the value placed on group identity over individual expression and also reflecting, to a certain extent, the cooperative nature of Balinese social organisation' (Gold 2005: 3–4). While noting that Javanese gamelan music is often considered as expressing not only the 'essence' of Javanese identity, but the 'way of being', Brinner warns against the idealization and simplification of this view, pointing out that cultural practices are influenced by a range of factors and can change over time (Brinner 1995).

The culture of playing

There are certain rules of behaviour around gamelan instruments, which all musicians observe. Shoes are removed before playing (as they are before entering a house or temple in Indonesia), and the instruments should not be touched with the feet and should not be stepped over. This breaks the connection between the instruments and the spirits, and the player must apologize to the instruments if this happens. Mallets should be placed on the instruments, not on the ground after playing. The spirit of the gamelan is thought to be embodied in the large gong, and offerings of flowers or food are often made to the gong before performances and on important days (Pickvance 2005).

One of the most important aspects of a gamelan performance is the ensemble feeling, the 'laya' (Tenzer 1998: 49). It is not considered enough to just play accurately; as there is no single conductor to watch who is giving these directions, as in a Western orchestra, the group has to feel and respond together to the speed-ups and slow-downs, and to sudden changes in dynamics. Similarly, gamelan playing does not allow for individual expression or overt displays of virtuosity; 'the ideal is the cultivation of absolute coordination and channelling of each member's artistic personality into a unified musical expression' (Tenzer 1998: 14).

The concept of 'Rasa' is important to gamelan playing. There are various translations of this word among scholars of gamelan music, such as 'feeling' (Walton 2007), 'musical affect' or 'emotion' (Benamou 2010) 'inner meaning' (Walton 2007) and 'mood' (Pickvance 2005). Pieces of music express different Rasa, and the musicians should convey these through their playing. Compositions can be categorized by their Rasa, which could include 'sad pieces, exuberant pieces, flirtatious pieces, and so forth' (Walton 2007: 35).

Relevance to music therapy

Considering the nature of gamelan music and instruments, several aspects are relevant to its potential use in music therapy practice. The communal nature of the music and the importance of cooperation and respect in playing may relate to therapeutic goals in group music therapy. The different moods or 'Rasa' of pieces and the different types and styles of gamelan, which express different cultures and temperaments, could all be employed for specific therapeutic purposes. The lack of a conductor emphasizes the need for listening to others, which may be a developmental skill being addressed in music therapy. The instruments, being pre-tuned and relatively simple to play initially, cater for a range of abilities and experience levels, which is also important in therapy settings.

Gamelan in the West

Gamelan has inspired and influenced many Western composers including Debussy, Messiaen, Britten and others. They have been impressed by its richness and complexity (Sorrell 1990) and have incorporated ideas to varying degrees in their compositions. Traditional gamelan music has been used widely in education; a major factor in its proliferation is a mention in the National Curriculum in the 1980s as an example of music from another culture that children should be taught about (Ruffer 1998). Since then, educators have emphasized its value in teaching basic musicianship and composition, and in giving an orchestral experience for children with a range of ability levels (Ruffer 1998; Mitchell 2000; Morrison 2007).

One of the earliest accounts of the use of gamelan with people who have special needs is given by ethnomusicologists Sanger and Kippen (1987), who report on an experiment to incorporate Balinese gamelan within an integrated summer music course for physically handicapped and able-bodied people. They found that social interaction was developed through musical interaction, and that the gamelan catered for all levels of ability, both musically and in terms of playing techniques and therefore offered possibilities and challenges to people with a range of abilities and disabilities.

Reports on the use of gamelan with people who have hearing impairments describe the benefits of it being a multi-sensory experience, the visual and tactile stimulation, the unusual sounds and tunings and the way the vibrations can be felt in different parts of the body (Palmer 1991, 1996; Smith 1997). Hawley (2005) notes that the music can be simplified without losing its connection to traditional music structures.

References to the use of gamelan with children and adults who have learning disabilities identify the importance of sensory aspects of the gamelan, and additionally stress its effectiveness in developing group interaction, reinforced by the fact that the gamelan is 'a family of instruments which belong to each other, rather than a haphazard mixture' (Crawford 1995: 5). Crawford further suggests that the gamelan should not be completely separated from its cultural context, which provides opportunities for using dance puppets and other artefacts.

The main research into the use of gamelan workshops for people with learning disabilities has been conducted by MacDonald with various collaborators, (MacDonald 1996; MacDonald, O'Donnell and Davies 1999; O'Donnell et al. 1999; MacDonald and Miell 2000, 2002). In these studies the authors show that taking part in gamelan workshops can improve the musical and communication skills of people with learning disabilities, and develop joint attention (MacDonald & Miell 2002). They conclude that there are many personal and social gains can be made from participating in this music, which in part stem from the structure of gamelan musical form and how one has to work as a group within it.

An expanding area of gamelan use is within the penal system and other secure settings. An ethnographic study of the Good Vibrations project, an organization that runs gamelan residencies in secure settings (Wilson & Logan 2006), demonstrated that prisoners found it beneficial in a range of ways, including as a way of getting to know and work with others, to feel part of something, to distract themselves and to be soothed by the music, and to help them gain confidence. The accessibility and alien nature of the gamelan were considered to be important to its success. Gamelan playing with female prisoners who self-harm was also found to have benefits, to reduce self-harming behaviour, and potentially to prepare participants for group therapy (Digard, von Sponeck & Liebling 2007). Mendonca (2010) emphasizes the 'socially transformative nature' of the Good Vibrations projects, both on individuals and on aspects of the institution.

Smaller research projects have suggested that playing Balinese gamelan can help children with attention disorders by improving their sense of timing and ability to manage their behaviour (O'Brien 2013). Gamelan listening was shown to reduce anxiety and physiological responses in patients with ventilator support in Indonesia, where familiarity with the music was thought to be a positive factor (Suhartini 2011).

Methodological considerations

There are several parts to this study that use characteristics of naturalistic enquiry, as defined by Lincoln and Guba (1985); it uses qualitative methods and has an emergent design – that is, the research design has unfolded through 'the interaction between inquirer and phenomena' as all elements could not be known beforehand – it uses purposive sampling to ensure the scope and range of data found is maximized, and has an inductive rather than reductive approach to the data analysis as this is 'more likely to identify the multiple realities to be found in those data' (Lincoln & Guba 1985: 40) The main sources for data collection in the study were the practice of gamelan playing, both in Indonesia and the West, and the practice of gamelan tutors who work with people who have special needs and special populations. Therefore, a naturalistic paradigm that used qualitative methods to gather data from natural settings was indicated.

In order to investigate current practice of using gamelan with special-needs groups and to identify therapeutic benefits and relevance to music therapy practice, the method of conducting semi-structured interviews with a purposive sample of gamelan tutors was chosen. The data analysis method of thematic analysis (Braun & Clarke 2006) was used to analyse transcriptions of these interviews. This is an inductive approach that generates a rich and detailed account of the data through the repeated coding of data and distillation of this into themes. A further layer of detail to the thematic analysis was generated through taking some of the themes generated from looking at the work of gamelan tutors into clinical music therapy practice. This would generate more information to take into the overall data synthesis and would provide more detail to be used in the development of guidelines for gamelan use in music therapy practice. In this part of the study therefore I moved into the role of practitioner–researcher and investigated my own practice of using gamelan in music therapy through the setting up and running of a series of music therapy sessions that used gamelan instruments, referred to as the School Project. I then returned to the role of researcher on completion of the project, and used the clinical data produced to evaluate the original themes and their relevance to music therapy practice.

Reflexivity

It is important in qualitative research to acknowledge and maintain awareness of the researcher's own position in relation to the phenomena being studied and the impact of self on the research. This relationship is one of the key features of naturalistic research that differentiates it from positivist approach, that 'the inquirer and the "object" of inquiry interact to influence one another; knower and known are inseparable' (Lincoln & Guba 1985: 37). Denscombe (2007) proposes there are two ways in which the researcher can deal with the involvement of self in qualitative research: by controlling their own values, beliefs and attitudes so that they remain detached from the production and analysis of data; or by acknowledging their involvement and 'the way their research agenda has been shaped by personal experiences and social backgrounds' (Denscombe 2007: 301). The position can then be taken that this involvement is actually a resource for the research rather than a limitation, and can be used to gain 'privileged insight' into the topic. As both a gamelan player and a music therapist, I have experience and opinions about both practices. I have strived to maintain a position between the two extremes described by Denscombe (2007) by acknowledging my involvement in both at all stages of the research, and considering reflexively whether these were informing or affecting decisions made in the research process and data analysis. By keeping the research questions in mind throughout the study and focusing only on the data relevant to this, I sought to minimize researcher bias and subjectivity. However, I recognize that the phenomena and experiences I have investigated are, as Wheeler and Kenny emphasize, 'seen through the researcher's eyes and heard through the researcher's ears and thus that they are shared through the researcher's voice' (Wheeler & Kenny 2005: 67). Therefore, it cannot be claimed that the study is entirely objective.

Ethical procedures

Ethical approval for the study was sought from Anglia Ruskin University using the Research Ethics Guidelines, which were applied for in two stages. The first was ethical approval for the overall study and for the interview procedures; this was obtained before commencing the study. The second part of the ethics application concerned the clinical project; as in this emergent design the participants for this aspect would not be known until the preceding parts of the study were completed, ethical approval for the clinical project was applied for once the participants had been chosen. This was granted before the clinical work commenced. A range of participant information sheets and consent forms were designed for the different groups of participants involved in the study – the gamelan tutors being interviewed, the school staff involved in the gamelan music therapy project, and the children and their parents or carers. The information sheets for children were written in simple, appropriate language and illustrated with pictures of the gamelan instruments.

The research study

Mapping exercise

To locate gamelan tutors I first conducted a mapping exercise to search for all gamelan sets and gamelan activity in the UK. About fifty contact addresses were initially found for gamelan sets; these were emailed with a short series of questions to answer, about gamelan work with participants who had special needs. From the replies received, twenty-five gamelan tutors were identified who had undertaken work of this nature. Fifteen of these participants felt their work was significant or recent enough to answer the series of questions. The replies received gave a broad picture of the work currently being undertaken in this area. Tutors were working with a wide range of participants in a variety of settings, including concert and orchestral centres, schools, arts centres, psychiatric hospitals and prisons. Most of their work was undertaken in one-off workshops with just a few tutors conducting week-long residencies. Participants for these workshops included adults and children with learning disabilities, physical disabilities and autism, adult and youth offenders, children with hearing or visual impairments, adults with mental health difficulties, and young adults with acquired brain injuries. The most commonly used type of gamelan was Central Javanese, with smaller numbers using Balinese or West Javanese. This exercise provided sufficient information to select a purposive sample of tutors to take part in the semi-structured interviews.

Semi-structured interviews

Nine gamelan tutors were selected for interview, who between them represented all the types of gamelan, participant groups and working practices identified in the mapping exercise. An interview schedule was developed from the themes identified through the literature review and the responses to the mapping email. This was first piloted, and the question areas were further refined. Tutors were invited to talk about a range of topics including their background and training, practical aspects of the work, aims and outcomes and their thoughts on the appeal of gamelan, its particular qualities and any therapeutic elements to gamelan playing. The interviews were transcribed and subjected to a thematic analysis. Six key themes were identified, relevant to the research question of what the therapeutic benefits of gamelan playing for people with special needs are. These were: accessible; encourages engagement; offers many group work possibilities; therapeutic effects; sensory range; and cultural heritage.

In addition, two further sets of themes were identified, Procedural themes and Tutor themes. The Procedural themes related to practical and factual information about the types of instruments and how sessions were run. These themes were relevant to the consideration of how music therapists could use gamelan in practice. The Tutor themes described the experience, training and approaches of the tutors, and the aims they had for this work. Following this, I considered the themes in relation to music therapy theory and practice and drew out the aspects that had most relevance to the main research question.

Clinical application of themes

In order to address the research question of 'How can music therapists use these benefits in clinical work in more depth and evaluate the relevance of the interview themes', I then set up and ran a short-term music therapy project using gamelan in a special school with children who have learning difficulties. The project was informed by the three sets of themes; I used a small selection of Balinese instruments to work with a pre-existing group of children, a form-group, and employed musical structures of traditional gamelan music and music therapy techniques. Several of the therapeutic aims of this work related to those identified as outcomes of gamelan playing: to help the pupils work together better as a group, to improve their attention and concentration, to develop their communication skills and to have an enjoyable music experience from which they could gain a sense of achievement. An evaluation of the work, conducted through a case study and interviews with the teaching assistants involved, demonstrated that the therapeutic group aims were largely achieved and several of the individual pupil aims were either fully or partially met. The three sets of themes were then reviewed again in relation to the music therapy project and the elements that were most relevant and useful for music therapy practice highlighted. The project demonstrated that gamelan playing could be used as a music therapy activity for this group of participants.

Research outcomes

In the final part of the study, the qualities and features of gamelan music and playing that have relevance for therapeutic use, which were identified through the literature and research review, were re-considered together with the themes identified through the analysis of the semi-structured interviews, and with the outcomes of the School Project. By reviewing all of these aspects, comparing and combining ideas, the specific features of gamelan music that are relevant to music therapy practice were defined.

Several of the identified features related to the nature of the instruments and to the music. Two of the outcomes were that clients will want to participate in playing, and that they will be able to do so. These could be considered the most fundamental; for therapeutic interactions to take place, clients need to be motivated to engage in playing and to be able to do so. Features such as the exoticness of the instruments and music, the visual and sensory appeal and the interesting sounds were shown to draw participants in and encourage engagement. The accessibility of the instruments, clear and adaptable playing actions and musical structures enabled people to have a successful playing experience quickly. Several of the identified outcomes were related to the group aspects of the music; that it is naturally a group-playing activity, and that within the music different levels of complexity and skills are required, making it accessible to participants with a range of abilities. The therapeutic outcomes of improving communication skills, due to the way the music works and the need to listen and respond to each other, are relevant to group music therapy aims. Because of the cyclical nature of the traditional music, and the possibilities it contains for simplification and adaptation, participants could experience increased self-confidence, self-esteem and have a sense of satisfaction through playing. The multi-sensory aspects of the instruments had relevance for many participants and improvements in mood and general wellbeing were also found to be benefits of playing. Other musical features were found that had relevance for therapy practice, which are beyond the scope of this chapter.

The identified features most directly related to culture were that gamelan playing has a cultural heritage that is useful for participants and for therapy, and that it can develop a sense of community among participants.

Cultural heritage

The relevance of cultural heritage was identified as a theme in the interview analysis and also in the literature and research projects examined, particularly in the work undertaken in prison settings. As shown in the ethnomusicology literature review, gamelan music conveys much of the values and societal ideals of the culture from which it comes. Brinner (1995) notes how both Javanese and Balinese gamelan music require community cooperation and harmony in the interactive musical exchanges, which are important aspects of these societies. Many of these values could be relevant in a therapy context and would be conveyed through the playing of traditional pieces, or simplified versions of them. The concepts of working as a group, helping each other and not standing out as an individual are important in both Indonesian society and in the music. They can also be aspects of music therapy work. Of relevance also is the concept of Rasa, the affect, mood or feeling conveyed in both the playing of and listening to gamelan music (Benamou 2010). This aspect of the music could be utilized in music therapy practice; specific pieces could be selected to help the group convey or explore particular emotions or dynamic qualities, as indicated by the therapeutic need. The choice of pieces according to their Rasa would, however, require further exploration, as the feelings assigned to pieces in Indonesia would not necessarily be recognized in the same way by non-Indonesian participants.

The cultural aspect within gamelan playing, which discourages individual free expression, could be contrary to therapeutic aims and therefore be seen as a disadvantage. However, a finding of the School Project was that it was possible to both allow and explore individual expression in gamelan-therapy sessions through adapting and combining music therapy techniques with gamelan-playing structures. This is also supported in discussions of the instruments by Walton (2007), who writes: 'The instruments in the gamelan are highly individual in timbre, range, rhythmic density and style, and the aim in ensemble playing is not a fusion of sounds, but the capacity for each instrument to retain its individuality in a group' (Walton 2007: 37).

In addition, the rituals surrounding gamelan playing were an important aspect identified by several gamelan tutors, both in the literature and the interview analysis, and endorsed in the School Project. While contributing to a sense of occasion for the playing, they too conveyed the values of respect, taking care and giving things worth, which were relevant to the participants and the therapeutic benefit of the sessions. The overall experience of playing something from a very different culture had a positive effect on participants.

Sense of community

Gamelan playing was shown to develop a sense of community among participants; the way traditional music works, and the egalitarian and inclusive aspects of playing, can lead to a strong sense of community in new and existing groups of participants. The interview analysis revealed a sub-theme, which is that the music is 'community generative'. This could have several uses within music therapy practice and, specifically, within a community music therapy approach, the gamelan could be used to develop a community, as a way for people to come together through an accessible, non-hierarchical musical activity.

The research findings demonstrate that there are many features of gamelan playing that make it an effective form of music for use in music therapy. A music therapist can take these features and use them intentionally for the purpose of addressing therapeutic aims within their clinical work. A further aspect of the study was to develop a set of principles for the use of gamelan in music therapy practice. These include the settings, instruments, musical structures, potential client groups and therapeutic aims that can be used in this work. Additionally, it is proposed that the music therapist should be experienced in gamelan playing and understand the associated culture, and that the culture and heritage should be retained and communicated in clinically appropriate ways. One outcome from the interview data analysis was that gamelan learning was more effective when it was linked to its cultural heritage. Being taught by a tutor who treated it as simply a set of instruments removed from its context was experienced more negatively than when this was included. Both the literature of gamelan and special needs and the interview analysis emphasized the importance of conveying the cultural aspects of the gamelan. This was also found to be important in the School Project. Cultural heritage can be transmitted through the music therapist's approach to the music and the instruments, how they conduct the session and the playing, the rituals and etiquette used, and the way the instruments are respected.

It is important to note that the 'foreign' aspects of the gamelan could be experienced negatively by participants, as was found in a small number of cases. For a few participants, something from such a different culture was viewed with suspicion. It suggested a non-Western culture, which had negative connotations for those particular participants; for others it was felt to be too different, and not relevant to their own lives and experience. A very few participants reacted negatively to the sounds of the gamelan. It is acknowledged that gamelan playing will not be suitable for everyone, and this needs to be taken into account when setting up music therapy work.

Conclusion

The study researched one non-Western musical tradition and found therapeutic relevance and applications for this. It follows that other non-Western musical traditions could have possibilities for therapeutic use. Further research into this is therefore indicated to develop music therapy theory and practice in this area. A recommendation of the study is that music therapists could benefit from learning about the music of other cultures, such as gamelan. It does not imply that therapists will only be able to work with Indonesian clients in this instance, but that by learning how to use the music of another culture they will extend their range of musical responses and become more open to listening to and incorporating other musical traditions in their playing.

The findings of the study can be generalized to a broad context. The research is based on literature and interviews that refer to work with a range of participant groups and settings; therefore, the list of gamelan features relevant to music therapy is applicable to this wide range of potential clients, settings and therapeutic purposes. Some examples of the potential use of gamelan include mental health, community, learning disability and family contexts. Regular group gamelan playing could be used in different mental health settings; for people with chronic mental health issues living in the community, gamelan playing could offer a consistent musical structure and opportunity for shared musical play through which a sense of community, belonging and ownership could develop. Within inpatient settings, open groups would be a way to engage people in a positive and meaningful activity, facilitating contact with others and affecting mood. The involvement of staff in these settings would enhance the gamelan group's contribution to the ward life and community. Gamelan could be very effective in work with learning disabled children and adults who have sensory impairments, in educational, residential and community settings. The specific visual, aural and tactile qualities of the instruments can be used to engage participants in music therapy activities. Therapeutic work with families, in which relationships between family members are being considered, could be addressed through small-group gamelan playing. The components required for this, such as listening and responding to each other, fitting interlocking parts together and taking different roles within the music, could address therapeutic aims.

This chapter has focused on aspects of the research findings relevant to the transposition of culture. To take this research further, some specific areas could be chosen to investigate; music therapy projects could be undertaken with different clients groups, and the outcomes analysed to investigate, for example, whether any features have particular relevance with different participants that could then be used in specific clinical settings, and whether any new unidentified features can be found.

Note

1   The Orff Instrumentarium consists of xylophones, metallophones (often tuned to modes or pentatonic scales), drums and other un-tuned percussion, recorders and stringed instruments (Orff, G. 1974).

Bibliography

Benamou, M. (2010), *Rasa: affect and intuition in Javanese musical aesthetics*, New York and Oxford: Oxford University.

Braun, V. & Clarke, V. (2006), 'Using thematic analysis in psychology', *Qualitative research in psychology*, 3 (2): 77–101.

Brinner, B. (1995), *Knowing Music, Making Music: Javanese gamelan and the theory of musical competence and interaction*, Chicago and London: University of Chicago.

Brinner, B. (2008), *Music in Central Java: Experiencing music, expressing culture*, New York and Oxford: Oxford University.

British Association for Music Therapy (2012), *British Association for Music Therapy: Fact Sheet*. Available online at: www.bamt.org (accessed 13 March 2014).

Bunt, L. & Hoskyns, S. (2002), *The Handbook of Music Therapy*, London: Routledge.

Chong, H.J. (2009), *Authenticity in Music Therapy, Voices: A World Forum for Music Therapy*. Available online at: www.voices.no/columnist/colchong010609.php (accessed 23 August 2010).

Chong, H.J. (2010), *Internationalization vs. Globalization of Music Therapy, Voices: A World Forum for Music Therapy*. Available online at: www.voices.no/columnist/colchong 030510.php (accessed 29 June 2010).

Crawford, S. (1995), 'Open arts in Belfast', *Seleh Notes*, 2 (3): 5.

Darnley-Smith, R. & Patey, H.M. (2003), *Music Therapy*, London: Sage.

Denscombe, M. (2007), *The Good Research Guide: for small-scale social research projects* (3rd edn.), Maidenhead: Open University.

Digard, L., von Sponeck, A.G. & Liebling, A. (2007), 'All together now: the therapeutic potential of a prison based music programme', *Prison Service Journal*, 170: 3–14.

Futamata, I. (2005), *Things Asian Music Therapists should Learn, Voices: A World Forum for Music Therapy*, Available online at: www.voices.no/mainissues/mi40005000 168.htm (accessed 23 August 2010).

Gold, L., R. (2005), *Music in Bali: experiencing music, expressing culture*, New York and Oxford: Oxford University.

Hawley, R. (2005), 'What does a sound look like?', *Seleh Notes*, 12 (2): 5.

Ingram, K. (1997), 'Unity in Diversity', *Seleh Notes*, 4 (2): 8.

Lincoln, Y.S. & Guba, E.G.(1985), *Naturalistic Inquiry*, California; London: Sage.

MacDonald, R.A.R. (1996), 'Structured music workshops for individuals with learning difficulties: an evaluation study', unpublished PhD thesis, University of Glasgow, 1996.

MacDonald, R.A.R. & Miell, D. (2000), 'Creativity and music education: the impact of social variables', *International Journal of Music Education*, 36: 58–68.

MacDonald, R.A.R. & Miell, D.(2002), Music for Individuals with Special Needs: a catalyst for developments in identity, communication and musical ability, in MacDonald, R.A.R., Hargreaves, D.J. & Miell, D. (eds.) (2002) *Musical Identities*, Oxford: Oxford University.

MacDonald, R.A.R., O'Donnell, P.J. & Davies, J.B. (1999), 'An empirical investigation into the effects of structured music workshops for individuals with intellectual disabilities', *Journal of Applied Research in Intellectual Disabilities*, 12 (3): 225–40.

Mendonca, M. (2010), 'Prison, music and the "rehabilitation revolution": the case of Good Vibrations', *Journal of Applied Arts in Health*, 1 (3): 295–307.

Mitchell, R. (2000), 'With a gong in my heart', *Times Educational Supplement*, 25 February 2000.

Moreno, J. (1988), 'Multicultural music therapy: the World Music connection', *Journal of Music Therapy*, XXV (1): 17–27.

Morrison, N. (2007), 'The Java sound of music', *Times Educational Supplement*, 2 March 2007.

O'Brien, J. (2013) *Power of Art: Can music help treat children with attention disorders?* Available online at: www.bbc.co.uk/news/magazine-21661689? (accessed 19 June 2013).

O'Donnell, P.J., MacDonald, R.A.R., Davies, J.B. & Dillon, T. (1999), 'Video Analysis of the Effects of Structured Music Workshops for Individuals with Learning Difficulties', in R.R. Pratt & D.E. Erdomnez Grocke (eds.) *MusicMedicine 3: Music Therapy and MusicMedicine, Expanding Horizons*, Melbourne: University of Melbourne.

Orff, G. (1980), *The Orff Music Therapy: active furthering of the development of the child*, London: Schott.

Palmer, R. (1991), 'Deaf gamelan workshops – a new approach to music', unpublished report: Dartington College of Arts.

Palmer, R. (1996), 'Feeling the vibrations', *Seleh Notes*, 3 (3): 7.

Pavlicevic, M. (1997), *Music Therapy in Context: music, meaning and relationship*, London: Jessica Kingsley.

Pickvance, R. (2005), *A Gamelan Manual: a player's guide to the Central Javanese gamelan*, London: Jaman Mas.

Ruffer, D. (1998), 'Gamelan in the National Curriculum', *Seleh Notes*, 5 (2): 4.

Sanger, A. & Kippen, J. (1987), 'Applied ethnomusicology: the use of Balinese gamelan in recreational and educational music therapy', *British Journal of Music Education*, 4 (1): 5–16.

Smith, M. (1997), 'Deafness in the music experience', *Seleh Notes*, 5 (1): 1.

Sorrell, N. (1990), *A Guide to the Gamelan*, London: Faber.

Spiller, H. (2008), *Focus: gamelan music of Indonesia* (2nd edn.) New York and London: Routledge.

Suhartini, S.K. (2011), 'Music and music intervention for therapeutic purposes in patients with ventilator support: gamelan music perspective', *Nurse Media Journal of Nursing*, 1 (1): 129–46.

Tenzer, M. (1998), *Balinese Music*, Hong Kong: Periplus Editions

Walton, S.P. 2007, 'Aesthetic and spiritual correlations in Javanese gamelan music', *Journal of Aesthetics and Art Criticism*, 65 (1): 31–41.

Wheeler, B.L. & Kenny, C. (2005), Principles of Qualitative Research, in B.L. Wheeler, (ed.) (2005), *Music Therapy Research*. (2nd edn.), Gilsum, NH: Barcelona.

Wilson, D. & Logan, M. (2006), *Breaking Down Walls – The Good Vibrations Project in Prison*, Report, Birmingham: Centre for Criminal Justice Policy and Research.

Part II

Intercultural practice guidelines and skills sharing

Chapter 6

Developing intercultural good practice guidelines in dramatherapy

Ditty Dokter

Introduction

At present there are no figures for dramatherapy clients from diverse backgrounds in the UK accessing dramatherapy. Some small pilots indicate that more black and ethnic minority clients may access dramatherapy than other psychological therapies (Dokter and Khasnavis 2008). Some dramatherapy intercultural practice by UK dramatherapists has been included in arts therapies edited volumes (Dokter 1998), a special issue of the *Dramatherapy* journal (Dokter 2007) or general-practice volumes (Casson 2004; Jennings 1997; Jones 2007; Leigh *et al.* 2012).

Worldwide intercultural practice by dramatherapists may incorporate initiating training outside their own cultural context (Landy 1997), or following up students' ability to practise when they have trained in a different context (Dokter 1993). Increasingly, practice examples are incorporated in general dramatherapy volumes, for example, those related to trauma (Sajnani & Johnson 2014). Publications are also starting to appear about the effect of colonization on dramatherapy/psychodrama development (Fonseca 2006; Massaro 2006).

Interculturality derives from the understanding that cultures thrive only in contact with other cultures, not in isolation (COE 2014). Intercultural (psycho)therapy is a term used in the UK context (Kareem & Littlewood 1992) to indicate the interactive element in cultural dynamics between the different parties involved in therapy. Cultural differences refer to variations in attitudes, values and perceptual constructs that result from different cultural experiences (Zane *et al.* 2004).

Intercultural practice may be difficult to generalize in dramatherapy, because the different theoretical models used by dramatherapists (Karkou and Sanderson 2006; Jones 2005) are mainly based on psychological and artistic theories. This creates a risk of white-European ethnocentricity, as it does for other forms of psychological therapy. Psychological and arts therapies recognize that members of various cultural and ethnic groups differ in psychologically meaningful ways (Hiscox & Calisch 1998). Intercultural psychotherapy research shows that the following within and between group difference variables affect heterogeneity:

country of origin; immigration history; place of residence urban/rural; motivation for migration; acculturation level; socio-economic level; English proficiency; ethnic identification and preferred language (McGoldrick *et al.* 2004).

Therapist and client background variables

In 2007 and 2015 the British Association of Dramatherapists (BADth) undertook a survey to monitor heterogeneity among dramatherapists. In 2007 this was to test the hypothesis that dramatherapists were mainly white, middle class, female and able-bodied, with possible diversity in relation to spirituality and sexual orientation. We wanted this to be a starting point to compare figures of therapist backgrounds to those of client backgrounds to check the possibility of client–therapist match and to ascertain the incidence of intercultural practice by dramatherapists. We also wanted a base point to be able to evaluate whether training was accessible to trainees from a range of backgrounds.

The survey was undertaken with the BADth Equality and Diversity Committee and was a part of data gathering for doctoral research (Dokter 2007). In 2015 the survey was simplified and repeated using Survey Monkey.

In 2007, 60 per cent of the membership who completed the hard copies of the questionnaire; in 2015, 51 per cent responded to Survey Monkey, a digital survey tool. The membership has doubled in that time, so it is impressive to see that the response rates remain high, survey response rates being notoriously low. Dramatherapy remains a female-dominated profession: in 2007, 84 per cent was female, 15 per cent male (1 per cent blank); in 2015, 83. 8 per cent were female and 16.1 per cent male. The age groups are evenly spread over five year age intervals, with smaller groupings in the early twenties and over sixties. Table 6.1 presents the breakdown of the 2007 and 2015 figures (in percentages) in the context of the census figures for England and Wales, where the majority of dramatherapists live and practice.

Regretfully, therapist language (first or multiple) was not included in either the 2007 or 2015 survey, and this remains an area for research development. Heterogeneity among dramatherapists in comparison to the UK population is reasonably represented, although particular cultural groups are absent or under represented, such as Asian, Islamic or Hindu therapists. Whether and how the absence of certain backgrounds affects clients, needs to be researched. Recent psychotherapy research into client–therapist match has not shown any effect on therapy outcome (Lambert 2013), but culturally adapted treatment forms, especially those using culturally appropriate metaphors, affect outcomes (Lambert 2013). Before addressing cultural adaptations, it is important to look at client backgrounds, to ascertain whether dramatherapists work with clients from heterogeneous cultural backgrounds.

Figures on client backgrounds are hard to obtain. I mentioned in the Introduction that individual case studies are available, and one small audit of

Table 6.1 Dramatherapist cultural-background survey

Ethnicity/cultural background	BADth 2007	BADth 2015	Office of National Statistics 2011
White	75	69.3	86
Black	Combined	2	3.3
Asian	Black/Asian/Mixed	1.06	7.5
Mixed	5	4.5	2.2
Working class	10	15.3	These categories are not used by the census, which uses employment patterns
Lower middle class	7	21.7	
Middle class	46.3	53.6	
Upper class	0	0.56	
Buddhist	4	5.7	0.4
Christian	30	28.8	59.3
Jewish	5	4.3	0.4
Humanist	-	10.8	—
No religion	28	35.3	25
Pagan	–	3.1	Combined in
Spiritualist	–	6.5	other total 0.4
Mixed spiritual adherence	29	–	0.04
Islam	–	–	4.8
Hindu	–	–	1.5
Sikh	–	–	0.8

dramatherapy clients (Dokter and Khasnavis 2008) showed a higher number of black and minority-ethnic client referrals to a dramatherapy department than for other psychological therapy departments in the Adult Mental Health Trust, a large National Health Service provider of inpatient and community services for people with mental health problems. The diversity of clients was in fact more on a par with the surrounding community than the Trust as a whole. The methodology of comparing client referral background data with that of Trust service users and the surrounding community via census figures is easily replicable. It does require dramatherapy department involvement for sufficient numbers to be monitored, which is becoming very difficult in an era of cuts and lone-working dramatherapists.

Another research methodology is therefore required to study cultural treatment adaptations. One such methodology is vignette research.

Vignette research methodology

The approach to research sought to combine the capacity of narrative vignettes to generate rich insights into therapeutic practice, with the use of the Internet to enable an enquiry with a geographically dispersed population of participants. The following contextualizes the innovative approach in relevant debates within the literature, identifying key challenges that the methodology sought to respond to.

Approach to data generation – debates and issues: vignettes

Vignettes used within research have been defined as written or recorded scenarios that aim to stimulate reflection or discussion about specific situations. The work, in part, responds to debates within the literature relating to the 'challenges' to qualitative researchers concerning the opportunities and 'false promises of internet technology' (Gajjala, Rybas & Altman 2008; Kien 2008, Tutt 2008).

The research method relates to aspects of these definitions of vignettes as stimulating reflection and analysis. The method aims to develop their potential in new ways to examine therapeutic practice in education. In contrast to the common approach identified by Jenkins *et al.* and Simon and Tierney, the use of vignettes is innovative in that:

• they are neither hypothetical nor provided by the researcher
• they explore the specific possibilities that Internet-based communicative analysis linked to vignettes could offer.

Approach to data generation – debates and issues: internet technology and divisions between online and offline domains

The work, in part, responds to debates within the literature relating to the 'challenges' to qualitative researchers concerning the opportunities and 'false promises of internet technology' (Gajjala, Rybas & Altman 2008; Kien 2008; Tutt 2008). Gajjala, Rybas and Altman (2008), for example, express the need for researchers to find innovative ways of enabling greater understanding of meaning-making within web-based qualitative research interactions. The methodology developed in the following research can be seen as a response to Kien's call for work that progresses researchers' encounter with 'the intersection of online and offline practices' (2008: 1106) and Tutt's concern that there is a division between online interaction and offline practices. The methodology discussed in this article proposes a connection between new media and methodology, which can be situated within such concerns about 'division' and the need to respond to technological advances as offering new opportunities.

The research methodology attempts to bring the specific potentials of narrative-based online communication in research into contact with understandings of professional practice of participants' work 'offline' in the field of therapy in educational settings. It responds to Gajjala, Rybas and Altman's (2008) challenge in its attention to the accounts of participants about their experience of communication and meaning-making within Internet-mediated communication within the research.

Benefits and limitations

The generation of data in the study aims to combine the *benefit* of a narrative vignette written by each therapist with a second element: the mutual analysis of the vignette narrative conducted through MSN Messenger and email between the therapist and the researchers. MSN Messenger was used, partly to explore the potential benefits of web-based ways of working outlined above, and partly as a way of dealing with the fact that participants were living far apart (Jones 2007; Mann & Stewart 2000).

It has been suggested that there are potential *limits* to the narrative vignette as a vehicle to engage in a meaningful way with the lived complexity of the processes and responses in the participants' experiences (Jenkins *et al.* 2010: 8). Vignette use can be critiqued for participant responses being conveyed through a 'normative screen', which 'minimises the potential' for feelings or issues that the participant may not wish to acknowledge to the researcher. He adds that another problem with vignettes is that they are a methodology that relies on memory and are 'therefore susceptible to memory impairment and retrospective reconstruction' (2008: 95).

Gajjala, Rybas and Altman (2008), in their research examining the production of cyber identities, argue the need for the field of qualitative enquiry to deepen its understanding of meaning-making and interaction in web-based relationships. The combination of documented conversation, further reflection on the conversation by email exchange and participant diary is a way to maximize the participant's opportunities to have their voice and 'vision' of their views and experiences included within the research's meaning-making of their work and to meet the 'need' articulated by Gajjala, Rybas and Altman. As the following analysis will show, the reflections of the participants on the research process were captured through the diary they kept, which provided insights into the meaning of the vignette, the process of the methodology and its perceived value to the researchers. Their inclusion aims to provide important perspectives and insight on the methodology.

Participants and procedure

Through an arts-therapy professional association (BADth), registered clinicians were offered the opportunity to be involved in the research, and sixteen therapists agreed to participate. Therapists had to be full members of BADth and practising in appropriate setting, as outlined above. Each therapist had to submit material from the setting confirming ethical clearance and that they complied with codes set by the Health Professions Council (HPC) Standards of Conduct, Performance and Ethics, Duties of Registrant (2003) (www.hpc-uk.org) and by the University's Faculty Research Ethics Committee.

Procedure and data generation: summary

The generation of data involved three elements. The first required the therapists to provide a vignette from their practice: a written description of a piece of clinical practice chosen by them to exemplify the ways they analysed their therapeutic practice. The second was a 'research conversation' using MSN Messenger and email. MSN Messenger was chosen as a mode of communication involving live, typed conversation, enabling immediate communication while keeping a record of that conversation for both parties.

Approach to data analysis: summary

The approach to the analysis of data drew on Elliott (2005), Riessman and Quinney (2005) and Robson (1993). They situate the process of analysis of narrative, qualitative research within hermeneutic or interpretive traditions. Riessman and Quinney's (2004) review of narrative approaches identifies standards for 'good' narrative research in relation to data collection and analysis. Their analysis focuses upon a 'comparative approach', which involves an examination of transcripts and the identification of similarities and differences among participants' narratives (Riessman & Quinney 2004: 404–5). The analysis drew on Elliott's (2005) and Robson's (1993) summary of approaches to drawing conclusions from qualitative narrative data: patterning though the noting of recurring themes; and clustering in the grouping of areas with similar charac-teristics, identifying variables including the examination of causal networks, along with the development of chains or webs of linkages between variables. The same approach was then taken in relation to the third element of data: the reflections on the research process by participants. Here, patterning, clustering, and the development of chains of linkages were also used to analyse the transcripts.

Previous intercultural vignette research had been undertaken in relation to populations inside and outside the UK (Colkett 2007; Sajnani 2010; Doonan 2007). Within the UK we received vignettes from sixteen dramatherapists, six of which were described as 'intercultural practice' and specifically mentioned the dynamics and ways of working in that context. In the following section I give two examples of these vignettes, one where the vignette and conversation are presented subsequently, and one where they are integrated. They give a flavour of the integration between the therapist-initiated vignette and the subse-quent research conversation.

Examples: two intercultural practice vignettes

Therapist vignette and research conversations: Lucy – intercultural adoption in a mixed heritage family

This vignette describes a dramatherapy intervention with an adoptive family of multiple heritage, living in a predominantly White English area.

The mother's heritage is African/Caribbean and the father's is Caucasian/Chinese and African/Caribbean (White English in appearance). Having two sons now fourteen and sixteen, they adopted Lucy (ten) – not her real name – at age nine months and, three years later, had a son, now seven. Lucy's heritage is English/Caribbean. The therapist is White English.

The goal was to secure the child's placement. Funding was for twenty sessions: ten hours of weekly direct work with the referred child and her parents; and a further ten hours with siblings and parents. The main problems prompting referral were:

1   Lucy's sexualized behaviour towards two of her three brothers and with younger children outside the family, which caused the family to feel isolated;
2   Lucy's intense jealousy of her younger brother; and
3   Lucy's unwillingness to talk, which created constant difficulties in communication.

A key aim of this intervention was to help Lucy understand why she was adopted. Lucy was placed for adoption when she was nine months old, from her (White English) foster carer where she had lived since three weeks of age. At birth, Lucy had suffered drug withdrawal, and spent her early weeks in an incubator. She was removed to foster care because her mother was drug-addicted, and often in prison for drug-related offences. Lucy had no relationship with her father, who was involved with her mother only briefly. Lucy has a (White English) half-sister, six years older, living with maternal grandparents who decided they were too old to take on Lucy as well. Lucy had grown up convinced her (white) mother and grandparents had given her up because she was 'black', despite her adoptive mother's attempts to explain this was not the case. Having experienced the humiliation of being treated 'differently', Lucy's adoptive mother recalled being followed by security men in stores, ignored in queues, and stared at threateningly. She had trained her children to 'rise above' racial taunts and worried that Lucy felt estranged from her family. It seemed likely that for Lucy the birth of her youngest brother in an adoptive family was confirmation that she was not 'good enough'.

THERAPEUTIC PLAY AS DESCRIBED BY THE THERAPIST

Although it was important to encourage Lucy to know about her history, we started with play as a way to build our relationship, to explore Lucy's perceptions and to observe her coping strategies. After selecting toy people and animals she placed in a sand tray, Lucy told the story of a *farmer* 'learning her lesson' from disguising herself as a *vet* as a cover, in order to exchange her *animals* for better ones owned by her kindly and successful *neighbour*. The therapist interpreted this metaphor that Lucy viewed herself as an 'impostor' in her family, where everyone else seemed 'better' than her. The story ended with the dishonest *farmer* admitting guilt (illustrative of Lucy's sense of self-blame) and the *neighbour* inviting collaboration so they became *friends*.

Each week, using toy people and animals, puppets, dolls, doll houses, clay and play dough, Lucy developed stories that revealed her anxiety about being perceived as predatory and her fear of uncontainable impulses. From creating her adoptive family, Lucy developed a story in clay in which she had each member enjoying an *adventure*, but she needed a lot of encouragement and persuasion to find any heroic role for herself, finally deciding she had the ability to 'calm *everyone down*'. Positively identifying with such a maternal role indicated that she wanted to model her adoptive mother. Lucy enjoyed this, and although her adoptive mother initially could not see the value, she appreciated it on being advised that having interested adults 'hang on' to the child's every word replicated the early attachment dance, which provides infants with vital social and cognitive information.

EXPLORING THE LIFE HISTORY

Towards the end of the first session, we read the history to acquaint Lucy with the facts I had gathered from her files, in response to which she told us she felt 'much better', as if something had changed. She regretted never having believed her adoptive parents' explanations. Each week we examined Lucy's life history, using such techniques as a life map of places she had lived and an exercise whereby water represented 'love' that *flowed* until *blocked* by 'suffering' (cling film). While sad to realize her birth mother had been addicted to drugs, Lucy was relieved to be told she wanted to keep her baby, but had simply not been able to look after someone else.

Over the third week, Lucy began speculating that her (birth) mother and grandmother were still yearning to see her. Dramatizing the story at this stage proved to be a most effective means for exploring Lucy's assumptions and fantasies. To help her gain a realistic picture, we enacted scenes in which I took the roles of *mother* and *grandmother;* Lucy's adoptive mother acted as *nurse, neighbour* and *social worker*. Lucy began to take such roles such as *police officer* and *Judge*, with us adults guiding her as to the conversations likely to have taken place. Hence, as *Judge*, Lucy interviewed her *birth mother* and *grandmother* and gained answers to her painful and difficult questions.

THERAPIST-PERCEIVED CHANGE AGENTS

Using a variety of materials for imaginative play, alongside focusing on the life history, empowered Lucy to find new ways of being and responding. Having felt unloved and excluded, the experience changed her self-perception to feeling wanted and entitled to membership of her adoptive family, all of whom report feeling more closely bonded. Lucy's, and her family's, heritage proved to be one dimension of a complex prism of issues, of which it was important for the therapist to be aware without being overly distracted from addressing the whole.

RESEARCHER–THERAPIST CONVERSATION EXCERPT

Researcher: I'm very interested in you saying, in the first stages in your work with Lucy – 'play as a way to build our relationship' – can you say a little more about that?

Therapist: Play and the five senses is the way that young children explore their world and relationships, therefore play is a more natural way to communicate with children than relying purely on verbal interviews. Having fun removes the pressure and allows children to express themselves through the privacy of metaphor, process experience, and show you how they feel and think. It may help you to know I have elaborated this in my book (Moore 2012).

Researcher: Can you say a little more about (i) how you considered Lucy used the five senses in her building a relationship with you, and (ii) how you handled your role in the play/five senses?

Therapist: Lucy played using figures in the sand tray (sense of touch), toys taking on 'role' (sights and sounds), moulding clay figures to develop stories (touch and smell – horse poo mentioned, etc.); also, using play dough, she made a selection of foods (taste by association), which were personified into a story of conflict (that was resolved).

I see my role as to reflect sensitively how things make me feel, to validate emerging feelings. I take the view that all the characters reflect aspects of the person and their preoccupations, and I aim to empower the child (as the character) to resolve matters for themselves. For example, in the vegetables story, I reflected how miserable Penny Peas must feel at being squashed by Peter Potato but notice that Peter Potato has few friends so perhaps he's lonely and jealous of Penny Peas, etc. It led to discussing what colours and smells remind us of – green/yellow – being sick, jealous, etc. I use water to symbolize love that flows until it gets blocked by hurt (represented by cling film). When the cup is sealed, nothing can pour in or out. It's a graphic way to show how love can be shared.

Researcher: I'm interested in the ways you look at change within your work here.

In the Outcome section you refer to ten sessions with siblings and parents together. I would be interested to hear how the dynamics changed with the siblings present?

Therapist: Actually, although funding allowed for this, I think I saw the two older brothers, together (without parents and sister) then the youngest with his sister and mum together. Lucy reacted as proud to include her brother in storytelling. I think it really helped to heal the divide and him to accept her more.

Researcher: Can you say a little about how you saw therapeutic change in relation to dramatizing the story, what did that offer Lucy?

Therapist: Lucy's assumptions were that she had been rejected and abandoned by her white mother because she was black. This was reinforced with grandparents not wanting her either, as they had her sister who was white. Her fantasy was that she was 'evil' probably reinforced before therapy on hearing she had been giving her parents and siblings 'evil looks'.

Researcher: How did this come out in the sessions with you/how did Lucy show this to you as a therapist – did she refer to it/narrate it, etc?

Therapist: It was based initially on info from the adoptive mother, and subsequently was apparent from the relief on the child's face on hearing my account of her life history and from the questions she asked the Judge and relatives in the drama.

Dramatizing her history helped her to know the full story of how things came about. Her adoptive mother taking part helped her see things through her child's eyes.

Researcher: What do you think the difference was for Lucy in engaging in this within drama as compared to being told it? And (ii) given that you were 'in role', too, how do you think of this – how do you think Lucy experienced this in terms of her relationships with adults from the past, say, and with you in the present as her therapist taking on a role alongside her adoptive mother?

Therapist: The difference is that walking the story, physically re-enacting it, she has to make decisions in role about how she reacts to others, including those who previously rejected her. She can change the outcome, get revenge, fictionally (stamp on model of abuser, etc.) and replaying it helps anaesthetize the pain, plus new memories are formed each time. In terms of my role, Lucy will experience someone being very interested in her reactions, replicating the mother/infant attachment dance via exaggerating things theatrically, comically, etc. The adoptive mother is encouraged to take helpful/rescuing roles (teacher, concerned neighbour, nurse, etc) and say things like 'this would never have happened if I'd been there – you'll be safe with me now!', etc.

VIGNETTE 2: NAOMI AND DAVID IN AN ADOLESCENT SCHOOL EXCLUSION UNIT

This is an integrated vignette and research conversation set in an educational exclusion unit in a metropolitan city.

Therapist vignette

Naomi, 15 years old, diagnosed with emotional and behavioural difficulties (EBD), had, for some weeks been demonstrating her conflicting feelings towards myself and the dramatherapy space. On the one hand, she would often recommend someone she termed 'naughty' to go to their session, giving a physical shove towards my room. On the other hand, she forbade me speaking in her presence, accidentally 'trod' on me, pushed me when passing and loudly told other staff how much she hated me. She had been to my room once and declared herself bored within five minutes, but checked out the space and equipment. Naomi mentioned she had spent hours on her own as a pre-school child with a computer screen for company.

Research conversation:

Researcher: How did you understand her ambivalence? What dramatherapy perspective did you use in the work?

Therapist: My sense of her had been as a very vulnerable person, who was just not going to show it. She had been very let down by her mother and that was ongoing. There was a little sister who was sweet and petite, who the mother kept calling up as an example. Naomi had clearly been neglected. She could not trust me, while she wanted the room and was fascinated. When she first came she liked playing with all the things, she said she was bored but she did not stop playing. This session shows how she found her way in. She brought her shield (David) and she created the session and interaction on her terms. Since, in this setting, I'd found textbook dramatherapy frequently rejected, I tried to maintain the possibility for play, however it may be presented. Following the theory of play and the acknowledgement of discrepant communication in Johnson's Developmental Transformations (2015), the following is an example of how therapist and space were used in a playful, exploratory way on the clients' own terms.

Therapist vignette:

One day, David, 16 yrs, wanted his hair woven by Naomi, who worked in a hairdressers at the weekends. David struggled with literacy and had already served a sentence for a stabbing. He had come occasionally for sessions before and enjoyed destroying things that could safely be destroyed.

Conversation

Researcher: Can you give me examples?
Therapist: I had a lot of cardboard boxes that could be cut/destroyed and soft
  toys that could be disembowelled.

Vignette continued

They announced they would be coming to my room that day. We agreed on
a time. This was going to be real not play hairdressing. Naomi had all her combs
and brushes in her bag. Afro-Caribbean hairdressing can take hours and
hairdressers are often culturally important meeting places with extended opening
times and a relaxed, family-friendly atmosphere. They arrived, arranged cushions
and chairs to create a comfortable, functional hairdressing corner and gave me
permission to sit nearby. Naomi declared the group an all-black one. I'm white,
Welsh, Naomi is from Sierra Leone and David is British with family from
Jamaica. They chatted as they might in the hairdressers. David asked for a mirror
in which he gazed fascinatedly throughout the session. My offers of roles and
scenarios were rejected.

Conversation continued

Researcher: What roles and scenarios did you offer?
Therapist: I offered to be someone else in the hairdresser (another customer,
  hairdresser, neighbour). This was rejected. They wanted a sort of net-
  curtain, a separation and I had the feeling that if I changed my role Naomi
  would have struggled even more with my presence. She was trying to work
  me out as myself, as a therapist. She wanted to me to stay put.
Researcher: Would you know if others who had wanted to come?
Therapist: She made it clear they would not be allowed that session.
Researcher: Was her saying it was a black group she said you were not in it?
Therapist: On the contrary, I was part of the group but Naomi feared I would
  align myself with the white students. She was banning them because she
  had chosen who would attend. I did feel privileged that I was allowed in
  this black group. My skin colour was permitted. She had quite a negative
  view of white people and I had been allowed in. They seemed to want
  me to be someone who attended to their needs and who understood I was
  to stop talking if I started 'chatting shit', (usually in connection with
  something emotionally charged).
Researcher: You were not allowed to ask about or comment on anything
  emotional?
Therapist: If I asked does your mum do your hair for example.

Vignette

Relaxed and comfortable, with each other for protection, they started to talk, with minimal prompting, about recent experiences.

Conversation

Researcher: Given the fact that you were not allowed anything emotional what sort of prompting?

Therapist: He was looking at his face and really enjoying what she was doing. I think I asked about school and their experiences at school. From that they discussed about being told they were naughty/bad from the word go. I probably asked if they remembered being small.

Researcher: That was allowed?

Therapist: That is the way, you throw them in, some get thrown back and some are allowed in.

Vignette

David had clearly been shaken by the violence he had encountered in prison and he showed me how many feet away from a murderer he had slept. He had been told he was a thug but saw a 'good' face in the mirror. Naomi talked despairingly about her home life and confusing relationship with her mother. At this point she showed me a sharp hair instrument and said I would feel it if I stepped out of line. She said she wished her skin was lighter, she wished she was not black. We talked about racism.

Conversation

Researcher: I wondered what sense you made of that interaction?

Therapist: From Naomi?

Researcher: At that point it is more a three-way conversation.

Therapist: Re David, he likes his face, is a handsome young man, he likes what he sees. But in contrast he is called a thug, got in trouble with the police and got branded. He was fourteen-years old at the time and he was absolutely terrified and somehow this happened, a sense of not getting his own life and how it turned out that way. He was definitely a victim too, more than once. And he was never aggressive to me, only to other pupils if they crossed him – he did not want them to get too close. Mostly though, people did not bother him. He got on well with the girls, partly because was good-looking – they wanted to mother him and he was a good friend. He could be trusted, I think.

Researcher: Re Naomi, David talks about being violent, a thug and then she threatens.

Therapist: Oh yeah, she was way more aggressive than him. She could not control herself and used her size to dominate.

Researcher: What do you think happened at that time for her to feel threatened, and threaten?

Therapist: Almost as if we were coming too close. The threat is about being vulnerable – the same applies – if you feel emotionally vulnerable you threaten. For her it is a logical solution /response. I think she felt she had removed her mask somewhat, and she had to be very careful about what I might do. If I did something wrong she might feel hurt and I needed to be controlled more so she could keep safe.

Vignette discussion re intercultural change agents in dramatherapy

In analysing the data from the vignette research the following change agents were highlighted. For Lucy in Vignette 1, it was important to work with her life story through metaphor, to explore her attachments. As a therapist, the awareness of and working with the systemic therapeutic relationship and the impact of racism were crucial.

For David and Naomi in Vignette 2 working through metaphor was still important, but for these adolescents, having choices in the therapeutic relationship with peer and therapist, working with dynamics of inclusion/exclusion in exploring power issues to address the effects of racism and social exclusion, were crucial.

Across all sixteen UK vignettes the main change agents across included working within a safe distance and 'allowance'. Therapists allow clients to play and try out new ways of being; clients allow themselves to play and try out new ways of being. An additional change factor is the opportunity to physically create and physically experience.

This vignette research is now followed up on different continents to compare/contrast therapist perceptions of change agents in dramatherapy and to identify cultural concepts influencing this perception.

International good practice guidelines

The British and American dramatherapy professional associations have been developing intercultural good practice and cultural competency guidelines and have engaged in a process of exchange in this development.

According to cultural competency models, (arts) psychotherapists must cultivate an awareness of their cultural identities and beliefs to better understand how their perspectives impact on their perceptions of their patient (Ponterotto *et al.* 2009). General awareness of one's values and attitudes is positively associated with how (arts) psychotherapists think about and behave with their patients, as well the strength of the therapeutic relationship.

Doctoral research into therapists' racial identity, with a particular emphasis on white identity, was undertaken by Tuckwell (2002). She identified four ways in which white identity may impact on transference issues, distinguishing between inter- and intra-ethnic (counter) transference:

- Inter-ethnic transference: overcompliance and friendliness; denial of ethnicity and culture; mistrust, suspicion and hostility; ambivalence
- Intra-ethnic transference: omniscient/omnipotent therapist; traitor, autoracist, ambivalence
- Inter-ethnic counter-transference: denial of ethnocultural differences; clinical anthropologist syndrome; guilt; pity; aggression; ambivalence
- Intra-ethnic counter-transference: overidentification; distancing; cultural myopia; ambivalence; anger; survivor's guilt; hope and despair
(Tuckwell 2002: 67–8)

The Equality and Diversity Committee of the British Association of Dramatherapists (www.badth.org.uk) has drafted guidelines that apply adaptations within the triangular transference (Jones 2005) as follows:

Medium: interventions focusing on cultural identity, verbal and non-verbal communication, body based, use of metaphor
Therapist: working alliance and safety, openness to explore therapist and client cultural identity, transparency and expectations, shame and oppression issues
Client: choice, transparency, disclosure and shame issues, issues about religion, working with interpreters

The North American Dramatherapy Association (www.nadta.org) have also gone through a process of consultation. They consulted cultural competency guidelines from the American Psychological Association (2002) and Art Therapy Association (2011), as well as the Association for Multicultural Counselling (1996), codes of ethics from the COE (2010) and the Canadian Music Therapy Association (1999).

NADTA are finalizing five guidelines (2015) to elicit further debate and exchange of good practice in the areas of:

1 commitment to cultural awareness and knowledge of self and others
2 commitment to cultural responsibility in dramatherapy practice
3 commitment to cultural responsibility in dramatherapy training
4 commitment to cultural responsibility in dramatherapy supervision
5 commitment to cultural responsibility in advocacy and organizational change.

Conclusion

This chapter gave examples of different research methodologies used to develop intercultural good practice, ranging from survey and audit to vignette methodology for more specific practice-based research about change agents and the development of intercultural good practice/multicultural competency guidelines.

Bibliography

American Art Therapy Association (2011), *Multicultural Competencies*. Available online at: www.arttherapy.org/upload/multyicultural_compentencies2011.pdf (accessed 14 August 2015).

American Psychological Association (2002), *Guidelines on Multicultural Education, Training, Research, Practice and Organisational Change for Psychologists*. Available online at: www.apa.org/pi/oema/resources/policy/multicultural-guidelines.aspx (accessed 17 April 2016).

Association for Multicultural Counselling and Development (1996), *Multicultural Competencies*. Available online at: www.multiculturalcounseling.org (accessed 17 April 2016).

British Association of Dramatherapists, *Draft Intercultural Good Practice Guidelines*. Available online at: www.badth.org.uk (members site) (accessed 14 August 2015).

Calisch, A.C. (1997), 'Multi Cultural Perspectives in Art Therapy Supervision', in R. Hiscox and A.C. Calisch (eds.) *Tapestry of Cultural Issues in Art Therapy*, London: Jessica Kingsley.

Canadian Association for Music Therapy Code of Ethics (1999). Available online at: www.musictherapy.ca (accessed 17 April 2016).

Casson, J. (2004), *Drama, Psychotherapy and Psychosis*, London: Routledge.

Colkett, D. (2007), [vignette], in P. Jones, *Drama as Therapy: Theory, practice and research (volume 1)*, London: Routledge.

Council of Europe (COE) (2014), *Intercultural City: Governance and policies for diverse communities*. Available online at: www.coe.int/t/dg4/cultureherotage/cities/Interculturality-en.p.l (accessed 28 October 2014).

Counselors for Social Justice (2010), *Code of Ethics*. Available online at: www.psysr.org/jsacp/Ibrahim_v3n2_1–21.pdf (accessed 14 August 2015).

Dokter, D. (1993), 'Dramatherapy in Europe – cultural contradictions', in Payne, H. (ed.) *Handbook of Inquiry in the Arts Therapies*, London: Jessica Kingsley.

Dokter, D. (ed.) (1998), *Arts Therapists, Refugees and Migrants reaching across borders*, London: Jessica Kingsley.

Dokter, D. (guest ed.) (2009), Special Intercultural practice Issue, *Dramatherapy*, 31 (2) Autumn 2009.

Dokter, D. & Khasnavis, R. (2008), 'Intercultural Supervision', in Jones, P. & Dokter, D. (eds.) *Supervision of Dramatherapy*, London: Routledge.

Doonan, R. (2007), [vignette], in P. Jones, *Drama as Therapy: Theory, practice and research (volume 1)*, London: Routledge.

Elliott, J. (2005), *Using Narrative in Social Research, Qualitative and Quantitative Approaches*. London: Sage.

Fonseca, J. (2006), 'The Roles of the Colonized and the Coloniser: in search of the identity of Brasilian psychodrama', in Figusch Z. (ed.) *Sambadrama*. London: Jessica Kingsley.

Gajjala, R., Rybas, N. & Altman, M. (2008), 'Racing and queering the interface: producing global/local cyberselves', *Qualitative Inquiry*, 14 (7): 1110–33.

Health Professions Council (2003). Available online at: www.hpc-uk.org (now Health and Care Professions Council (HCPC) (accessed 14 August 2015).

Hiscox, A.R. & Calisch, A.C. (eds.) (1997), *Tapestry of Cultural Issues in Art Therapy*, London: Jessica Kingsley.

Jenkins, N., Bloor, M., Fischer, J., Berney, L. & Neale, J. (2010), 'Putting it in context: the use of vignettes in qualitative interviewing', *Qualitative Research*, 10 (2): 175–98.

Jennings, S. (1997), *Dramatherapy Theory and Practice 3*, London: Routledge.

Johnson, D.R. (2015), *Developmental transformations: towards the body as presence*. Available online at: www.academia.edu/1795111/Developmental_transformations_Towards_the_body_as_presence (accessed 26 July 2015).

Jones, P. (2005), *The Arts Therapies. a revolution in health care*. London: Routledge.

Jones, P. (2007), *Dramatherapy Theory, Practice and Research* (2nd edn.), London: Routledge.

Jones, P. (2009), 'Vignette research in dramatherapy', *European Journal of Psychotherapy and Counselling* 11 (3): 251–66.

Kareem, J. & Littlewood, R. (eds.) (1992), *Intercultural Therapy: Themes, Interpretations and Practice*, Oxford: Blackwell.

Karkou, V. & Sanderson. P. (2006), *Arts Therapies: A Research Based Map of the Field*, London: Elsevier Health Science.

Kien, G. (2008), 'Technography, technology & ethnography – an introduction', *Qualitative Inquiry*, 14 (7): 1110–33.

Lambert, M. (ed.) (2013), *Garfield and Bergin's Handbook of Psychotherapy and Behaviour Change*, (6th edn.) New York: John Wiley & Sons.

Landy, R. (1997), 'Dramatherapy in Taiwan', *The Arts in Psychotherapy* 24 (2): 159–72.

Leigh, L., Gersch, I., Dix, A. & Haythorne, D. (eds.) (2012), *Dramatherapy with Children and Young People in Schools*, London: Routledge.

McGoldrick, M., Giordano, J. & Garcia-Preto, N. (eds.) (2005), *Ethnicity and Family Therapy* (3rd edn.), New York: Guilford.

Mann, C. & Stewart. F. (2000), *Internet Communication and Qualitative Research: A handbook for researching online*, London: Sage.

Massaro, J. (2006), 'The Roles of the Colonized and the Coloniser: In search of the identity of Brasilian psychodrama', in Figusch Z. (ed.) *Sambadrama*, London: Jessica Kingsley.

Moore, J. (2012), 'Theatre of attachment', *Adoption & Fostering Journal*, 30 (2):64–73. Available online at: www.researchgate.net/publication/233712168_percent27Theatre_of_Attachmentpercent27_Using_drama_to_facilitate_attachment_in_adoption (accessed 14 August 2015).

North American Dramatherapy Association (2015), *Guidelines of Cultural Response/Ability in Training, Research, Practice, Supervision, Advocacy and Organisational Change*. Available online at: www.nadta.org (accessed 14 August 2015).

Office of National Statistics (2011), *Census*. Available online at: www.ons.gov.uk/ons/guide-method/census/2011/index.html (accessed 14 August 2015).

Ponterotto, J.G., Casas, J.M. & Suzuki, L. (2009), *Handbook of Multi Cultural Counseling* (3rd edn.), London: Sage.

Riessman, C.K. & Quinney, L. (2005), 'Narrative in social work: a critical review', *Qualitative Social Work*, 4 (4): 391–412.

Robson, C. (1993), *Real World Research*, Oxford: Blackwell.

Sajnani, N. (2010), 'Mind the gap: facilitating transformative witnessing among audience', in Jones P. (ed.) *Drama as Therapy (Volume 2)*, London: Routledge.

Sajnani, N. & Johnson, D. (eds.) (2014), *Trauma Informed Dramatherapy: transforming clinics, classrooms and communities*. Springfield: Charles C. Thomas.

Tuckwell, G. (2002), *Racial Identity, White Counselors and Therapists*, Buckingham: Open University.

Tutt, D. (2008), 'Where the interaction is collisions of the situated and mediated in living room interactions', *Qualitative Inquiry*, 14: 1157.

Zane, N., Nagayama Hall, G.C., Sue, S., Young, K. & Nunez, J. (2004), 'Research on Culturally Diverse Populations', in M. Lambert (ed.), *Bergin & Garfield's Handbook of Psychotherapy and Behaviour Change* (5th edn.), New York: John Wiley & Sons.

Chapter 7

Intercultural skill-sharing in music therapy

Alexia Quin and Cathy Rowland

In many countries, music therapy is a recognized clinical discipline, with well-evidenced benefits to people with disabilities, emotional difficulties, mental health difficulties and a wide variety of special needs (Dileo Maranto 1993).

Nordoff-Robbins Music Therapy, Analytical Music Therapy, Benenzon Music Therapy, The Bonny Method of Guided Imagery and Music and Behavioural Music Therapy represent the 'Five International Models of Music Therapy Practice', which were defined and presented at the 1999 World Congress in Washington DC To contemporize this list we might add Neurologic Music Therapy (Hurt-Thaut & Johnson, 2015) and Community Music Therapy (Stige, Ansdell, Elefant & Pavlicevic, 2010). There is great variety within these different ways of working with regard to the emphasis placed on active participation, receptive (listening) techniques and improvisation, as well as differences in the music therapist's role. What they do all have in common is the underlying belief in the power of music to affect us at a deep level, regardless of illness or disability (Dasgupta & Majumdar, 2014; Aigen, 2014; Baker & Wigram, 2004).

Bunt and Stige suggest music therapy is now a truly international practice, with developments in South America, Africa, Asia and Australia as vital as those in the United States and Europe (2014).

The United States was the first country to develop music therapy as a modern profession and discipline and its first professional association was founded in 1950 (National Association of Music Therapy (NAMT)). There are now eight professional associations in North America, twenty in South America and two in Canada (Tsiris 2014). The UK professional body was founded over 25 years later (Association for Professional Music Therapists) and now there are sixty-one music therapy associations across Europe, some more focused on professionalization than others, sometimes more than one in any particular country. The location of world congresses over the years is also inspiring: Paris, Buenos Aires, Puerto Rico, Genoa, Rio de Janeiro, Vitoria-Gasteiz, Hamburg, Washington, DC, Oxford, Brisbane, Seoul and Krems, with over 1,200 music therapists, trainers, researchers and students from forty-six different countries presenting. But what happens if we look beyond capital cities or economically successful countries within any particular continent? In these places, music therapy remains in its infancy, largely reliant on dedicated pioneers sourcing information and ad hoc training from places where it is a more established form of intervention. As well as local pioneers, there are plenty of documented examples of contributors who have been music therapists travelling to other countries and undertaking clinical work beyond their own culture (Pavlicevic 1994; McInerney 1997; Cronly 1996; Bolger 2012). In such writing, focus is often given to a therapist's personal experiences of working in a culture that is not their own (Hadley & Hunt 2013), the fact that they are working in a context where the fit of their own training needs careful consideration (Salcin-Watts 2008), or in circumstances that bring particular local challenges or where the clinical focus has arisen as a result of local conflict (Storsve, Westby & Ruud 2010; Bergmann 2002). However, for some music therapists, their roles have not simply been that of clinicians, but as trainers seeking to leave a legacy with local people so that the benefits of music therapy can continue beyond their time in the field (Wells 2008; Rickson 2009; Coombes 2011; Margetts, Wallace & Young 2013; Navarro Wagner 2014; Parker & Younes 2014). A much smaller sample have considered the role of music therapy within the wider sphere of international development (Heidenreich 2005; Bolger & Skewes 2013).

Some exploration of the impact of skill sharing over time has been undertaken by other arts therapies (Kalmanovitz and Lloyd 2005; Jennings 2011). However, there is little written in the field of music therapy, and little that attempts to quantify the impact of such work. Such writing could elicit findings that could helpfully inform future intercultural skill-sharing initiatives as music therapists continue to consider their roles beyond the traditional clinical space.

Since 1995, the British charity *Music as Therapy International* has been providing introductory training to local care staff, teachers, physiotherapists, speech therapists and psychologists (our Local Partners) working in just these places. As an established organization focusing purely on this role, in contrast to individuals working in isolation, *Music as Therapy International* has the infrastructure to both deliver, evaluate and strategically review its activities across different geographical regions. Growing demand for the charity's projects internationally (to date it has delivered thirty projects to care settings world-wide), requests for consultancy from music therapists in the UK and beyond and its strong presence within Index of International Music Therapy Organisations suggests the organization is well placed to undertake research that could inform future intercultural practice.

Music as Therapy International's roots lie in Romania, and grew from Quin's experiences of volunteering in an orphanage in the early 1990s. At this time, Romania was a country heavily scarred by the tyranny of a dictator who destroyed freedom of thought among its people, ruined the country's economy and – perhaps most notoriously – devastated the lives of thousands of disabled children, who he separated from society and for whom he failed to provide care (Galloway & Wylie 1991). Quin was among the international volunteers who flocked to try to help. However, she quickly began to question this approach, and to identify the potential value of training local people, rather than relying on international volunteers.

In a pilot project designed in response to her first experiences in Romania, Quin invited the Irish music therapist Úna McInerney to spend 6 weeks working alongside local staff in an institution for children with complex needs compounded by lifelong institutionalization in the north of Romania, supported by Quin (Cronly 1996; McInerney 1997).

Twenty years later, the charity's core activity remains the provision of this introductory training through the delivery of skill-sharing projects to help our Local Partners improve the quality of life for marginalized children and adults with a range of disabilities. The charity does this by responding to requests from schools, hospitals, day centres and other care settings around the world. It then undertakes a feasibility study to identify the readiness of the Local Partner for a skill-sharing project and compatibility between them and the charity's approach. A training project is then designed, tailored to local need, before a volunteer team is recruited. The teams typically comprise one music therapist with relevant clinical experience and one 'assistant', who is interested to learn about music therapy alongside the Local Partners and will support the therapist in delivering the project. After an intensive induction provided by the charity in the UK and the host country, this team will live and work alongside the local staff for the duration of the project, work together to find ways to build a therapeutic music programme into the existing activities for the clients, to demonstrate how to run music sessions and to support the local staff – our Local Partners – as they try the new techniques themselves.

Following introductory training, the charity remains alongside our Local Partners, albeit at a distance. We recognize the challenges of pioneering new ways of working, and of the context and the clients with whom they work. Regular steering group meetings are held for each region, in which the charity works so the longer-term impact of projects, the strengths and vulnerabilities of the Local Partners are constantly reviewed and used to inform further support activities. These may include: requesting written reports to encourage reflective practice; returning to observe sessions and guide Local Partners in recognizing their successes as well as thinking about the challenges to their practice; facilitating peer-to-peer learning through the creation of a newsletter or online forum; targeted additional training focusing on clinical challenges or specific client groups; musical resources; local and national conferences; Skype and online supervision. We are proud that these support activities have enabled our Local Partners in Romania to maintain their music programmes for as long as 16 years. In addition to supporting our Local Partners in maintaining their work with music, the charity has also supported their development as 'trainers'. As well as sharing their music skills with their colleagues creating a so-called 'second' or even 'third' generation of practitioners, some have shared their practice more widely. Since 2010, one team has run twelve trainings in five different locations. Another is now working in partnership with the local educational inspectorate to roll out trainings in their local schools. Our most prolific trainer has trained over 1500 practitioners.

With the emergence of our Local Partners as trainers we started to question the long-term impact of our skill-sharing projects: Which skills did staff adopt and develop readily? Which skills were more challenging to acquire and use independently? Were skills overlooked when Local Partners trained others (a Chinese Whispers effect)? Just as the charity encourages reflective practice among its Local Partners, it applies the same paradigm to its own work. This led to the creation of steering groups for each region and the appointment of an Advisory Panel of Music Therapists, who have a strategic role within the charity. The involvement of many of these people led to the creation of the Competency Framework, an evaluation tool that summarizes the skills required to deliver music sessions informed by key principles of music therapy. This tool is now integral to our assessment of our Local Partners' skill-base, helping us to quantify practice strengths, but also to identify training needs. It also serves to evaluate the longer-term impact of the charity's work.

After 10 years of delivering multiple projects within Romania, and in response to local requests, the charity took the decision to extend its work into other countries. We recognized that our approach would need to be carefully tailored to each new region, but we needed to be confident that our projects retained the necessary constants to achieve the lasting impact seen in Romania, in other countries. To identify these constants, a working party from the charity reviewed previous projects to identify their shared qualities and key features. This enabled us to distil our approach into four core values, which now underpin all our projects and remain heavily informed by Quin's original motivation to set up the charity:

> *Sustainability*: Every Music as Therapy International project aims to have an impact that lasts longer than our active presence within the participating community. We believe effective partnerships between employees, volunteers and Local Partners are fundamental to sustainability. We make every effort to enable Local Partners to build on our investments in their communities. We share our resources with others working in related fields to broaden the impact of our work.

> *Integrity*: We are honest and ethical in all that we do and engage in responsible decision-making that reflects the highest standards of conduct. This ensures that our credibility, leadership and use of charitable funds are never in question. We demonstrate best practice at all times, guided by a professional code of ethics.

> *Respect*: We are passionate about understanding the real needs of communities we work in and believe sensitivity to local culture and customs

are vital. Time allowed to listen to, observe and learn from our Local Partners is integral to our projects. A collaborative approach is paramount.

Innovation: Making concepts of music therapy accessible to people in non-traditional contexts requires creativity, compromise and vision. We encourage innovative practice to achieve this and strive for continuous organizational development as we learn from each project.

(Music as Therapy International/About us/Our Values Webpage)

The music therapists who are recruited to lead these projects have varied in their training backgrounds and prior experiences. They are given autonomy, with guidance available if required, to choose their approach and which skills they share with their Local Partners. Despite this freedom, all projects have ultimately drawn on the UK model of improvisational music therapy. The late British Music Therapist Tony Wigram describes the many clinical applications arising from this model, where both client and therapist improvise music together (Wigram 2004). In our own literature we describe the model in very clear terms:

[T]he use of music and sound in a structured setting to promote the mental, physical, emotional and social well-being of an individual . . . [The] music is used initially to establish a point of contact with the child or adult and then as a means of addressing, within a safe, secure environment, whatever difficulties the child/adult is experiencing. For example, it may be used with children who are withdrawn and unresponsive to draw them into shared musical activity. It can equally be used to channel – in a positive and constructive way – the energies of very active individuals.

(McInerney & Quin 1995)

Within the UK model of improvisational music therapy, a further two key principles have been fundamental to the approach shared by all our music therapists:

1   A person-centred approach, informed by the work of the humanistic psychologist, Carl Rogers (Rogers 1951, revised 2005).
2   A secure attachment base, as originally described by John Bowlby (Bowlby 1951, revised 2005).

When demonstrating a person-centred approach, our therapists have often emphasized Carl Rogers's Unconditional Positive Regard, defined by Rogers as a basic acceptance and support of someone regardless of how they present themselves. This is further informed by Daniel Stern's Affect Attunement (Stern 1985). Affect Attunement also provides a tangible tool for creating a secure attachment with the children and adults with whom our international partners work. Both of these key principles are modelled through the use of structured activities and free improvisation, offering children and adults opportunities for musical interaction (Streeter 2001), non-verbal self-expression, and the development of social skills and creativity (Oldfield and Bean 2001; Hadley *et al.* 2011).

One distinct difference between the UK model of music therapy from which we draw and the cross-cultural training we provide – by which we mean training within which there is interaction between two or more cultures – is the emphasis on musical skills: In the UK, music therapists are required to be professional standard musicians, with many having undertaken music degrees prior to completing their postgraduate music therapy training. In contrast, we demand no prior musical training of our Local Partners. This may explain that while some bravely develop their abilities to improvise with musical instruments and their voices, the majority favour structured activities and pre-composed songs. These are therefore given more focus during our skill-sharing projects than they might be given during music therapy training here in the UK. Interestingly, our Local Partners often request additional training in musical skills once the more generic techniques are well established in their work. It is as if taking a person-centred approach and focusing on creating a secure attachment base is sufficient for achieving immediate and impactful changes to practice. Once our Local Partners are confident with these two principles, they become eager to develop their music-making in order to build on these foundations.

At this point it should be made absolutely clear that, while it is helpful to draw comparisons between the focus of music therapy training and our skill-sharing projects, our projects do not attempt to train people to become music therapists. This is made explicit to all participants, and heavily informs the emotional level at which our therapists explore music-making with our Local Partners and their clients. Not only would it be impossible to cover all the teaching requirements of clinical training within the scope of our projects, but it would also require screening of participant local practitioners and thus create a barrier to access. We prioritize enhancing the existing workforce's skills, and many people we work with would not have the musical or academic skills to be able to complete the full training. Nor might it be what is needed or wanted locally. Additionally, attempting to create therapists could risk unsafe practice, given a lack of supervision available locally.

To date our projects have taken us to Romania, the Occupied Palestinian Territories, Rwanda, Peru, Georgia, Myanmar and back to the UK. Wherever we have worked, these core values and theoretical basis have proven to be culturally relevant, albeit it with careful tailoring to suit local strengths and needs. To achieve this, the charity and its volunteers work hard to identify and align their approach with the cultural norms of project countries: '. . . the cultural characteristics of a particular group, that is, the norms, values, attitudes, and behaviours that are typical of an ethnic group and that stem from a common culture of origin transmitted across generations' (Phinney 1996). Furthermore, we recognize the sub-cultures that exist: the (sub-) cultural norms that distinguish a rural village from a country as a whole, a marginalized group of disabled children from the wider village, a room of children within an institution from the whole community on site. All of this aligns with our Core Value of 'Respect'.

The ways in which our core values translate into our cross-cultural skill-sharing approach can be shown in the following very different initiatives:

Distance Learning Programme: Changes in the structure of care settings in Romania and advances in technology have given us the opportunity to adapt our *in situ* skill-sharing model to enable distance learning. Our Distance Learning Programme, for people working with young children with disabilities in Romania (Hadley, Lovell, Quin & Rowland 2010, revised 2013) has been designed to teach practitioners (usually teachers, careworkers and psychologists) how to develop their own music programmes with children with special needs under the age of ten. It offers monthly online tutorials, supported by a face-to-face teaching weekend, culminating with an eight-week practical assignment. Following each tutorial, students submit written assignments and are supported through their practical work with online supervision. The programme has now been running for four years and has produced many highly skilled practitioners who continue to develop their own programmes within their own workplaces. We are currently looking at ways it can be rolled out to benefit people working in other countries, piloting its use in the Occupied Palestinian Territories in 2015.

Training DVD: When considering how to support local practice in culturally meaningful ways we created a training DVD for our Local Partners in Rwanda. We were aware that written resources and email or Skype support was difficult for our Local Partners, due to low literacy levels and minimal access to the necessary technology, or even a local postal system. They themselves had said they thought it would be helpful to have a film they could refer to, in order to refresh their understanding of techniques or to re-focus their work. The DVD was produced in French and English with Kinyarwandan subtitles and the majority of footage was of our Local Partners themselves working. We strove to keep the cross-cultural distractions to a minimum, to use the film to showcase the skills of the staff, provide a way to share good practice and to create something that could be used as a training tool for new staff too (Anderson, Haire & Quin, 2013).

Training for Trainers: When considering how we could help our Local Partners continue using their new skills, after our training team had left, and developing their approach over time, we developed the 'Training for Trainers' course to support peer-to-peer skill sharing, and further build local capacity. Thirty Local Partners from across Romania have attended this course, which equipped potential trainers with the necessary knowledge and skills to teach others how to set up and run their own client-centred music programmes. Graduates were subsequently given a comprehensive Training Manual. Those who used this as a basis to produce their own locally led training courses, have been awarded a kite mark from the charity and have rolled out training courses throughout Romania and beyond.

Having discussed the approach of the charity and the scope of its work, we turn now to the question of evaluation. This is undoubtedly important in these outcomes-focused times, but also as a tool for strong reflective practice and, when sensitively undertaken, a supportive process for the evaluated person. Evaluation of all our international projects and wealth of support activities in the form of feedback questionnaires has given us much qualitative evidence. The sample below gives a flavour of their appreciation for the difference that our input has made to their working lives.

For one Local Partner in Rwanda, a country where disabled people can still be extremely marginalized, our project had enabled her to see her clients differently: 'For music therapy I received many skills and I thank you so much because you helped me to discover different ways in communicating with mentally challenged people'.

Similarly, for Local Partners in Beit Sahour and Romania, it seems that our projects had given them completely new insights and skills:

> We have so many trainings as teachers, and they are all about the teacher – the planning, the lesson, the thinking, the materials – but this training was the first one that taught us how to be with children, to communicate with them, be with them and help them be more confident . . . It is like a mother and baby, who can talk without using words.
>
> (Local Partner, Beit Sahour 2010)

> I am delighted that music therapy has given Carmen the opportunity to express her emotions, her thoughts, and that it has given me the opportunity to get to know her in a way that I haven't managed to in any other activities.
>
> (Local Partner, Romania 2005)

Additionally, we are aware that the long-term support has been valued and viewed as important by our Local Partners, such as Aura, a care professional in Romania, who wrote to us saying,

> I continued this work because I was supported by our trainers for 12 years. The musical instruments that helped me carry out the work were donated by Music as Therapy International. The continuous effort done by both

parties made this collaboration sustainable over time and helped us give sense to the life of abandoned people that didn't have any hope of someone reaching out to them.

(May 2012)

Despite this wealth of evidence from our Local Partners about the impact of skill sharing, it felt important that we should examine this more systematically. Follow-up visits had frequently confirmed that skills sharing had had a short-term impact, but what was the longer-term impact on those trained in the past? Was it true that intercultural skills sharing could provide an innovative and longer-term means of meeting the needs of vulnerable communities? If this was indeed the case, which were the skills which could be taught successfully by UK trained music therapists to those without a musical or therapeutic background and were there any limitations to this approach?

In order to see for ourselves the effects of the charity's intercultural skills sharing we decided to undertake field trips to carry out observations of our Local Partners' work. In September 2013, two teams of therapists visited nineteen settings in Romania and in 2012 and 2013, music therapists visited Rwanda and Palestine, (see Table 7.1). During each of these visits, which lasted a week, the therapists observed Local Partners' music sessions. The table below presents these visits within the context of the charity's history of skills sharing where, between 1995 and 2010, the focus was solely on skills sharing in Romania. As is shown, the Romanian Local Partners visited in nineteen settings had been trained over a fifteen-year period and some of them had received additional training and support. In contrast, the Rwandan and Palestinian Local Partners had each received a recent, single training project with no additional training. These variables, together with a multitude of others – national and local cultural differences, occupational status of Local Partners, length of training, as well as the presence of different trainers – suggest that any comparison of data arising from such visits, to be presented in the following section, would be extremely complex and therefore beyond the scope of this chapter.

In all locations, the observations of Local Partners' music sessions were carried out using the same evaluation tool, the Interactive Music-Making (music as therapy) Competency Framework. Originally conceived and devised by Hadley and Quin (2002), this tool was subsequently developed by Reynolds, Birnstingl and Robbie Mitchell (2013) and edited into its current full form by Hadley and Quin in 2012. It comprises four main elements, containing a total of five core competencies and thirty-five additional competencies, varying in complexity from basic practicalities through to techniques used to provide flexible emotional support. A sample of competencies is included in the table below under each other the elements. Each competency based on key concepts (shown in italics) is carefully defined through supporting information.

Table 7.1 Background information relevant to each field trip

Country visited	Rwanda territories	Occupied Palestinian	Romania
Therapists and observer(s)	Nicky Haire Caroline Anderson	Liz Coombes	Cathy Rowland Alexia Quin Hannah Hulin Becca Sayers
No. of Local Partners observed	3	2	18
Roles of Local Partners	Care worker/ activity leader	Teacher/social worker psychologist/ activity leader	Teacher/educator/ care workers/
Observation setting	2 day centre/ residential care setting	1 school	19 schools/day centres/residential care settings
Dates of training received by Local Partners.	2010	2012	1995–2006
Skill-sharing model(s)	• 6-week training project • Follow-up visit	• 6-week training project • Follow-up visit • Additional training • Distance learning programme • Tailored support activities	• 6-week training project • Follow-up visit
No. of original trainers	2	2	28

The purpose of the Competency Framework within this research was to provide a standardized tool to enable us to assess the extent to which skills from the initial training have been assimilated by their Local Partners.

In each geographical location, all therapists were aware of the multi-layered sensitivities around the process of ethical observation. In the nineteen Romanian locations visited by the authors within the short time span, visits to each site usually lasted between 2 to 6 hours, allowing minimal time to create a rapport with Local Partners as well as offer them ongoing clinical support. Furthermore, we were acutely aware of the potential conflict that becoming 'evaluator' may create with our previous roles as supportive mentors.

We were mindful that giving ourselves an overt authority status might feed into the traditional hierarchical systems that had historically been the norm in our Local Partners' workplaces, thus undermining the relationships carefully nurtured over the years. For these reasons we decided to observe only those

Table 7.2 Sample competencies from each element

Element 1:	The use of sound and music to develop interaction with a focus on interpersonal connections.
Example competency:	The practitioner follows the *child's initiation*, waiting to allow time to assimilate the *child's responses*.
Element 2:	The use of Interactive Music-Making principles to assess children, formulate goals and evaluate progress.
Example competency:	The *method* and progress towards the *individualized goals* is *evaluated* and *Interactive Music-Making (music as therapy) activities* are modified in accordance with the changing strengths and needs of the child.
Element 3:	An informed attitude and approach to working with clients with special needs.
Example competency:	The practitioner *takes responsibility* for the personal and physical safety of self and the client.
Element 4:	A confident use of musical skills and instruments with a focus on interpersonal connections.
Example competency:	The practitioner is able to *improvise simple songs* which reflect and are supportive of the child's responses.

Local Partners who stated they were comfortable to be observed. Even then, we took an ethical decision, when planning our visits, not to refer to evaluation as a secondary purpose of our observations, so as not to jeopardize the first of giving clinical support. By enabling our Local Partners, whether newly trained or experienced in using music programmes to opt into this process, conducted within time-limited supportive visits, it was possible to respect the sensitivities involved, while seeing for ourselves the impact of our skill sharing.

The findings that we will present in this chapter can therefore be viewed within a research design based on phenomenological hermeneutics. While phenomenology can be defined as the study of 'phenomena', the appearance of things as they appear to our experience, hermeneutics is understood as a theory of text interpretation. Phenomenological hermeneutics is therefore the study of text as live phenomena (www.phenomenologyonline.com/inquiry/orientations-in-phenomenology/hermeneutical-phenomenology/website). Drawing on this research design, we used the dynamic process of reflection, description, and interpretation based on live events, (our Local Partners' sessions), to convert our observations into the findings we present below. Our findings, therefore, originate from observation of live music sessions run by those Local Partners who had consented to being observed by us. The main elements of their approach were reviewed immediately afterwards through the lens of the Competency Framework. Subsequent reflections and discussions of these live sessions, leading to the collation and presentation of our findings, we suggest, can be viewed as a reading of 'text' in a phenomenological sense.

In order to ensure a clear, consistent reading of the 'text', other considerations were factored into our research design. First, videos from each of the five music therapists involved in these observations were viewed by a member of the *Music as Therapy International* team and scores checked to eliminate subjectivity.

Second, we decided to limit our interpretation of 'text' purely to what it revealed about the successes or limitations of skills sharing. As we have already demonstrated, the variance within our sample goes beyond differences of country or culture. There are considerations of sample size from each region, how skills were shared, how much experience Local Partners have since acquired, differences in role and professional status etc. Any ethical reading of 'text' or reflections upon our findings would need to take account of these – something that is beyond the scope of this research.

In order to prevent any comparison across the three localities, and ensure an ethical reading of text, we present our data fully anonymized. The four graphs below show the ranges in competence observed in our Local Partners across the following categories: client-centred practice, creating a secure attachment base, simple musical skills, and sustainable approach to practice.

Each category was broken down into a range of defined competencies drawn from the Competency Framework with each of the twenty-three participating Local Partners' practice graded as shown in Table 7.3.

As described earlier in this chapter, these evaluations can be viewed through the lens of phenomenological hermeneutics as a 'reading of text' – the text being a live event. All evaluations therefore were undertaken following live sessions. Prior to each field trip, training was given to evaluators to ensure that all ethical considerations for our Local Partners were maintained. The training also promoted a consistent approach across the evaluators – combining sharp observation skills focusing primarily on the core competencies with an intuitive sense of a Local Partner's overall skill level. These observations were recorded on a check list immediately after the 'event'. Although the viewing of videos by a second person ensured most reliable 'reading of text' we are aware that complete objectivity of these data could not be expected. We recognize that from a single, live event of a session, it was not always possible for every competency to be assessed and those that could be were inevitably based on memory recall, albeit recent.

The findings below are presented in four categories: client-centred practice, secure attachment base, sustainability and musical skills. The first two of these assess Local Partners' skills that directly reflect the theoretical basis of the training they have received, as outlined earlier in this chapter. The third category, 'A Sustainable Approach to Practice' reflects the charity's underlying core values of empowering its Local Partners and thus Local Partners' capacities to assimilate their training into their daily working lives. All three categories comprise groups of relevant performance criteria derived from Elements 1 to 3 of the Competency Framework. The fourth category, 'musical skills', comprises all performance criteria in Element 4 of the Competency Framework,

Table 7.3 Table showing the competency range achievable

80–100%	Very highly competent practice: The Local Partner demonstrated outstanding competence, which is completely consistent and embedded into their skills set
60–79%	Highly competent practice: The Local Partner demonstrated complete competence, or competence which was consistent throughout the observation
40–59%	Competent practice: The Local Partner demonstrated considerable competence, but exceptions were observed which suggest that this is not completely consistent
20–39%	Partially competent practice: The Local Partner demonstrated partial competence; for example, more than once, but not yet in a consistent way.
0–19%	Very partially competent practice: The Local Partner has demonstrated only fleeting or very partial competence, or demonstrated this competence in its entirety but only in a fleeting way, with no sense of repetition or consistency.

and reflects the creative medium upon which the training is based and shows the extent of skills acquired.

Each of the forty competencies within each of the four elements was considered integral to client-centred practice. As shown in Figure 7.1 the mean scores suggest that Local Partners demonstrated highly competent practice and that no Local Partners demonstrated less than the middle level of competent practice.

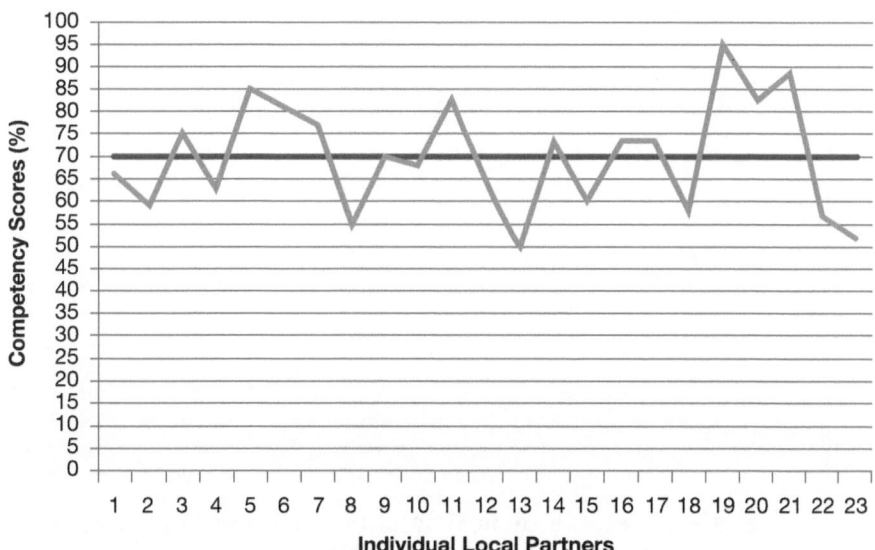

Figure 7.1 Client-centred practice

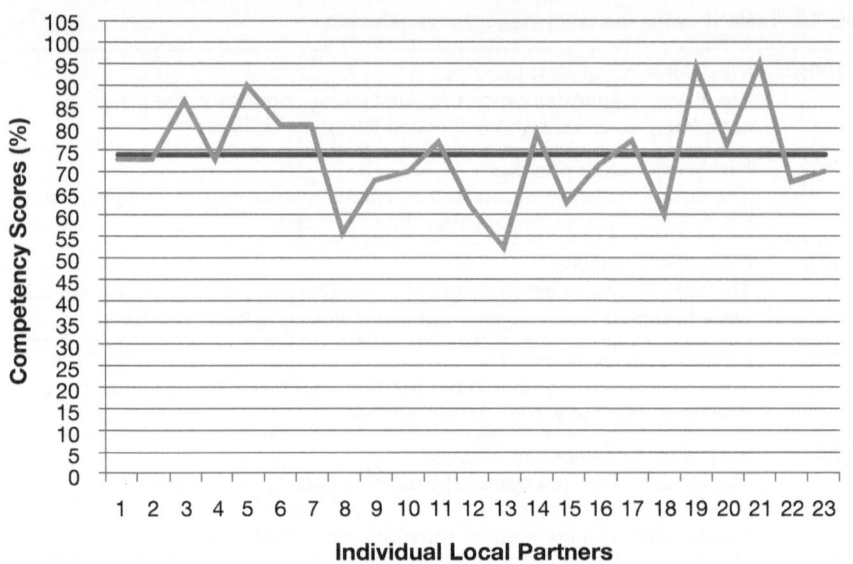

Figure 7.2 Creating a secure attachment base

We identified twenty-three competencies from the Competency Framework as integral to creating a secure attachment base. Again, the mean score demonstrated highly competent practice, with 48 per cent of Local Partners demonstrating higher than average competence in this category.

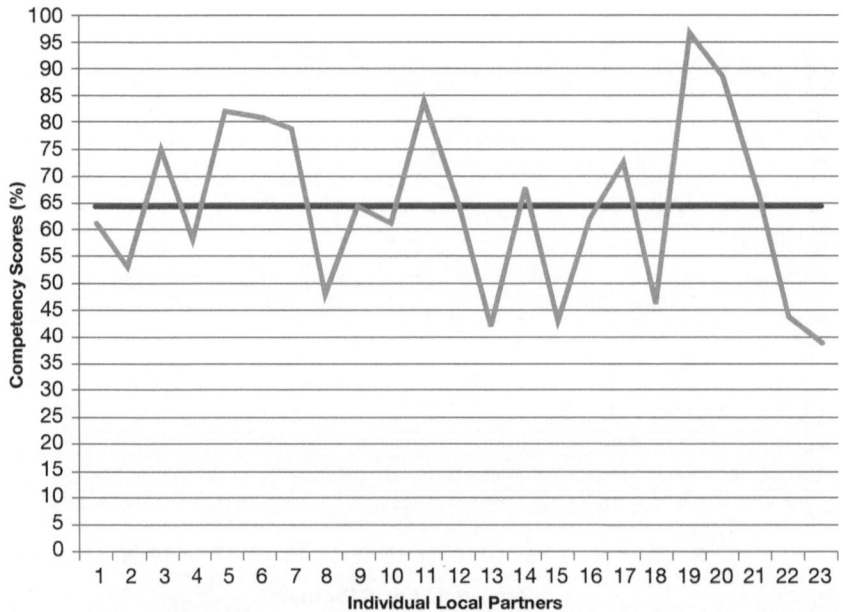

Figure 7.3 Musical skills

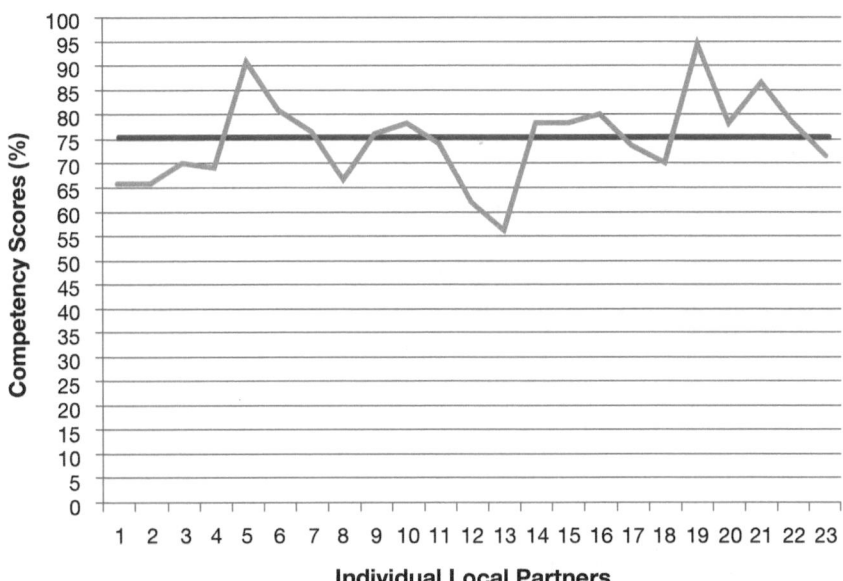

Figure 7.4 A sustainable approach to practice

Twenty-two distinct competencies were evaluated here to identify competence in using basic musical skills. These ranged from very simple skills, such as ability to use pitch, rhythm or to play simple percussion instruments, to more immediate skills such as being able to offer a flexible musical response, or to sing a simple song. To accommodate those few Local Partners with musical training, this element also assesses more advanced skills, such as the use of musical themes or harmony. The strong variance in these data reflects the disparity of musical confidence between our Local Partners: some considered themselves unmusical and were initially disbelieving of their musical potential; in contrast others brought prior studies of musical instruments, experience of church singing or participation in other culturally defined musical activities.

The charity's commitment to locally sustainable practice is reflected in the high average score achieved by participating Local Partners (75 per cent) evaluated across twelve relevant competencies.

As discussed earlier in the chapter, variance within the sample of participating Local Partners is a significant limitation to this piece of research. It is clear that more structured research would be necessary to truly extrapolate the multiple factors that influence the success of intercultural skill sharing. However, the Competency Framework served as an effective tool to identify where similarities did exist: in three categories (client-centred practice, creating a secure attachment base and a sustainable approach to practice). A reading of the data suggests that every Local Partner demonstrated skills that at the very least could be considered 'competent' according to our criteria. Variability in these data also indicates high or very high competence from some Local Partners. In the simple musical skills category, competence was indicated all round, except for one Local Partner and in this category also, high competence and very high competence were also present.

The range of individual scorings shown within the category of 'Client-Centred Practice' reflects some observations during our visits where a Local Partner's behavioural or educational approach took slight precedence over more therapeutic aims promoting spontaneity or individuality. Overall, however, these findings provide concrete evidence that intercultural skill sharing can effectively promote client-centred practice.

Although we have chosen not to interpret the data, by comparing competency trends between countries it is interesting to separate out our findings for our Romanian Local Partners against the category 'Sustainable Practice'. Their mean score indicates a high competence and that sustainability is sufficiently embedded into their practice. This is significant, because some of them have been running sessions for as long as 18 years, so it is a skill set that has been effectively maintained over time.

Although the scores from our other Local Partners in this category are also at the upper end of highly competent practice, we are aware how challenging it can be to maintain a music practice over the longer term. Perhaps our findings suggest that intercultural skill sharing can establish sustainable practice. What remains to be seen is whether or not this lasts the test of time in more than one country. The charity will continue to extend its portfolio of support activities to more recent skill-sharing participants, and we would therefore be interested to re-evaluate the extent of sustainable practice in these localities in five years time.

Prior musical training is not required of Local Partners before they embark on skill sharing with Music as Therapy International, but we wanted our evaluation to reflect the fact that we are training our Local Partners to use *music* as a form of communication. It is, perhaps, unsurprising, that for most of our Local Partners, this was their lowest scoring category. When reviewing our data, we noted the very high scores from two of our three Rwandan Local Partners, which indicated very highly competent practice, particularly within the simple music category. This pointed to something potentially significant, given the strong tradition of communal music-making within Rwandan society.

We are aware that our score for our Palestinian Local Partners of partial competence may not represent their true abilities. Their musical heritage is based on Arabic scales, rather than Western diatonicism in which the Competency Framework is rooted, and it rarely includes harmony and chords.

As their musical tradition is exceptional among our current Local Partners, it was valuable for us to learn that some of the musical skills we had identified within this section of our Competency Framework may need cross-cultural adaptation. In addition to the variables discussed in this chapter, we are aware of a possible substrata of other variables, which make it difficult to compare like for like. These include the culture of a staff team and perceptions of music sessions within the setting, the degree of management support for music sessions, staff sickness levels, work stress, professional status, degree of staff turnover within a setting, as well as wider socio-political or economic factors and their impact upon a setting. This multitude of variables mean that it is not possible to draw any valid conclusions relating to cultural influences over the impact of intercultural skill sharing with regard to promoting the use of simple musical skills.

The field visits undertaken by *Music as Therapy International* representatives in 2013–14 afforded an exciting opportunity to quantify the impact of intercultural skill sharing undertaken by music therapists. We acknowledge that due to the ethical nature of its design, this research is limited by its sample sizes, which are formed from self-selecting groups. We cannot therefore claim that our findings are truly representative of *all* the Local Partners we have trained over the last 20 years. Our research was also limited by the number of variables within the different sample groups, which remained too complex and multi-faceted to extrapolate.

In our view, however, the consistently high scores across all four categories from our samples, (albeit from a self-selecting group) provided evidence that aspects of the UK improvisational model of music therapy can be taught through skill sharing; they can be embraced cross-culturally by people with a variety of backgrounds, working in diverse places. It gave heartening affirmation to the fact that safe practice is both achievable and sustainable, with no Local Partner demonstrating incompetent practice in any area. While we acknowledge the sample was self-selecting and only confident partners may have opted in to observation visits, it is significant that there were no observed Local Partners unconscious of poor practice.

To examine the specific impact of intercultural skills sharing we suggest that further research based on a phenomenological, hermeneutic research design would be required. This would involve longer field visits than were carried out by the evaluation team, leading to the gathering of more data via quantitative and qualitative research methods, (structured interviews, questionnaires, additional observations). Consideration could be given to making the evaluation tool more user-friendly. We are aware of the high number of performance criteria in each element. While we consider each one valid in itself, we acknowledge that used within the context of a 'live event' such as a session, their relatively high number within this tool may pose challenges for the evaluator. Should further research be undertaken, we would consider streamlining this tool – perhaps by identifying and focusing more upon core skills to be assessed within each of the four categories. We believe this would in turn assuage any risk that the extent to which Local Partners were comprehensively evaluated might be influenced by the experience of the evaluator implementing the Competency Framework.

Interpretation of 'text' – of live interviews, conveying Local Partners' lived experience, supported by further session observations, would give a much fuller picture of the intercultural nature of skill sharing. Further extrapolation of some of the variables in subsequent findings may also be possible – for example, comparing the effectiveness of skills sharing among different occupational groups within the same setting. Careful consideration would still be needed if meaningful cross-cultural comparison were to be attempted.

In the meantime, we believe that this study represents a new, exciting step in intercultural music therapy research. It is hoped that this should encourage music therapists to continue to explore their role beyond the traditional clinic space and within the sphere of international development.

Bibliography

Aigen, K. (2014), 'Music-centred dimensions of Nordoff-Robbins music therapy', *Music Therapy Perspectives*, 32 (1): 18–29.

Anderson, C., Haire, N. & Quin, A. (2013), *Using Music with People with Disabilities* [DVD], London: Music as Therapy International.

Baker, F. & Wigram, T. (2004), 'The immediate and long term effects of singing on the mood states of people with traumatic brain injury', *British Journal of Music Therapy*, 18 (2): 55–64.

Bergmann, K. (2002), 'The sound of trauma: music therapy in a post-war environment', *The Australia Journal of Music Therapy*, 13: 3–16.

Bolger, L. (2012), 'Music therapy and international development in action and reflection: a case study of a women's music group in rural Bangladesh', *The Australia Journal of Music Therapy*, 23: 22–41.

Bolger, L. & Skewes, K. (2013), 'Demonstrating Sustainability in the Practices of Music Therapists: Reflections from Bangladesh', *Voices: A World Forum for Music Therapy*, vol. 13, no. 2. ISSN 1504–1611. Available online at: https://voices.no/index.php/voices/article/view/715/603 (accessed 3 Nov. 2014).

Bowlby, J. (2005), *A Secure Base: Clinical Applications of Attachment Theory* (2nd edn), London: Routledge Classics.

Coombes, E. (2011), 'Project Bethlehem – training educators and health workers in the therapeutic use of music in the West Bank', *Voices: A World Forum for Music Therapy*, 11 (1). Available online at: https://voices.no/index.php/voices/article/view/291 (accessed 3 November 2014).

Cronly, A. (1996), 'Music Therapy in Northern Romania: Work Experience, Documentation and Future Plans', unpublished Dissertation University of Exeter (see also Quin).

Dasgupta, S. & Majumdar, G. (2014), *Classical Music, Eastern and Western, as Therapy*, World Congress of Music Therapy.

Dileo Maranto, C. (1993), *Music Therapy: International Perspectives*, Pennsylvania: Jeffrey.

Galloway, G. & Wylie, B. (1991), *Downfall: Fall Of Ceaucescus and the Romanian Revolution*, London: Sphere.

Hadley, S. & Hunt, M. (2013), *Changing Levels of Comfort: Living and Working in Different Communities, Experiencing Race as a Music Therapist*, New Braunfels, TX: Barcelona.

Hadley, S., Lovell, E., Quin, A. & Rowland, C. (2010; 2013), *Music as Therapy for Young Children with Disabilities: A Distance Learning Programme*, London: Music as Therapy International.

Hadley, S., Quin, A., Mitchell, L. Reynolds, C., Robbie, J. & Rowland, C. (2002; 2005; 2013), 'Interactive Music-Making (music as therapy) Competency Framework', in S. Hadley & A. Quin (eds.), *Music as Therapy International*, London: Music as Therapy.

Heidenreich, V. (2005), 'Music therapy in war-effected areas', *International Journal of Mental Health, Psychosocial Work & Counselling in Areas of Armed Conflict*, 3 (2): 129–34.

Hurt-Thaut, C. P. & Johnson, S. B. (2015), 'Neurologic Music Therapy', in Wheeler, B. (ed.) *Music Therapy Handbook*, New York: Guilford.

Jennings, S. (2011), *Healthy Attachments and Neuro-Dramatic-Play*, London: Jessica Kingsley.

Kalmanovitz, D. & Lloyd, B. (2005), *Art Therapy and Political Violence: With Art, Without Illusion*, London: Routledge.

McInerney, Ú. (1997), *Cross-Cultural Music Therapy with Institutionalised Children in Romania: Music Therapy across Cultures*, British Society for Music Therapy Conference Papers.

McInerney, Ú. & Quin, A. (1995), *Music as Therapy for Children Ionaseni Project Booklet*, London: Music as Therapy International.

Margetts, L., Wallace, H. & Young, E. (2013), 'A potential space: approaching "outsider research" with classroom practitioners working with children with complex needs in Belarus', *British Journal of Music Therapy*, 27 (2): 6–23.

Navarro Wagner, A. (2014), 'Re-Framing Experiences in Gulu's Socio-Cultural Context: A Comt Point Of View', unpublished paper presented at the World Congress of Music Therapy, Krems.

Oldfield, A. & Bean, J. (2001), *Pied Piper: Musical Activities to Develop Basic Skills*, London: Jessica Kingsley.

Organisational values for Music as Therapy International. Available online at: www.musicastherapy.org/about_us/our_values.html (accessed 11 December 2014).

Parker, D. & Younes, L. (2014), 'Music And Resilience: Introducing Music Therapy in The Refugee Camps Of Lebanon', unpublished paper presented at the World Congress of Music Therapy, Krems.

Pavlicevic, M. (1994), 'Between chaos and creativity: music therapy with "traumatised" children in South Africa', *Journal of British Music Therapy*, 8 (2): 4–9.

Phinney, J. S. (1996), 'When we talk about American ethnic groups, what do we mean?' *American Psychologist*, 51 (9): 918–27.

Rickson, D. (2009), 'The use of music to facilitate learning and development in a school in Thailand: an exploratory case study', *The New Zealand Journal of Music Therapy*, 7: 61–87.

Rogers, C. (2005), *Client-centred Therapy: Its Current Practice Implications and Theory*, London: Constable and Robinson.

Salcin-Watts, E. (2008), *Transferring Music Therapy Practice into Non-Western Settings: Cultural Considerations and Reflections, New Ways of Serving Communities at Home and Abroad: A Resource Pack* (pp. 43–7), London: Music as Therapy International.

Stern, D. N. (1985), *The Interpersonal World of the Infant: A View from Psychoanalysis and Developmental Psychology*, London: Karnac.

Stige, B., Ansdell, G., Elefant, C. & Pavlicevic, M. (2010), *Where Music Helps: Community Music Therapy in Action and Reflection*, Surrey: Ashgate.

Storsve, V., Westby, I. A., & Ruud, E. (2010), 'Hope and Recognition: A Music Project among Youth in a Palestinian Refugee Camp', *Voices: A World Forum for Music Therapy*, 10 (1). Available online at: https://voices.no/index.php/voices/article/view/158/246 (accessed 18 April 2016).

Streeter, E. (2001), *Making Music with the Young Child with Special Needs: A Guide for Parents*, New York: Jessica Kingsley.

Tsiris, G. (2014), International Index of Music Therapy Organisations (IIMTO) (2nd edn.). Available online by Nordoff-Robbins at: www.nordoff-robbins.org.uk (accessed 2 April 2015).

Wells, M. (2008), Clinical Vignette, in *New Ways of Serving Communities at Home and Abroad: A Resource Pack*, London: Music as Therapy International.

Wigram, T. (2004), *Improvisation: Methods and Techniques for Music Therapy Clinicians, Educators and Students*, New York: Jessica Kingsley.

Part III

Ethnographic voices

Chapter 8

Voices within intercultural arts psychotherapy research and practice

An ethnographic approach

Allison Singer, Bojana Skorc and Vesna Ognenovic

Introduction

This chapter is based on ethnographic research that was undertaken in Serbia between September 2001 and September 2002, shortly after the end of the war in former Yugoslavia. The research concerned the use of dance and movement in psychosocial work with Serbian refugees and internally displaced (IDP) children and their families. The research centred on a Serbian non-governmental organization (NGO) called Zdravo Da Ste, also known as Hi Neighbour.

Zdravo Da Ste was founded by a group of Serbian psychologists and academics in 1991 at the beginning of the war in former Yugoslavia in response to the influx of refugee people. Their central concern was for the welfare of the refugee children. Zdravo Da Ste stated that their main aims were 'protecting and promoting development during war and post-war crisis . . . [and] provid[ing] . . . support in building social communities' (Zdravo Da Ste 2006). They described the activities in which they were involved as psychosocial support, cultural and social integration, professional training and skills development, income generating programmes, summer and winter camps for children, exhibitions, humanitarian assistance, etno[1] programmes and intercultural exchange. By the time I came to the field, Zdravo Da Ste had seventeen teams working throughout Serbia and Republika Srpska. My fieldwork was based with the Belgrade team, especifically with the children's team.

I chose to work with Zdravo Da Ste because I wanted to understand what the local people who had experienced the war considered important in their work with the arriving refugee people, rather than working with the interpretations of the international community. The methodology I used for the research integrated Dance Ethnography and DMP; I adopted a reflexive, feminist, applied anthropological approach. As in contemporary approaches towards Dance Anthropology and Dance Ethnography, my research was concerned with movement and other arts media including story, visual arts and etno as symbolic action; and the processes that generate, and the meanings behind, this action (Sklar 2001; Ness 1992). Within my research I used participant observation, including fieldnotes, formal and informal interviews, video and photographic documentation and journals. I also studied the Serbian written and spoken language, and began to learn about etno dance and music. It is important to note that I am a practising DMP and Dramatherapist as well as being a Dance Ethnographer and Ethnomusicologist, and the integration of these theories and methods informed all aspects of my research.

This chapter juxtaposes my methodology and understanding of the field with Zdravo Da Ste's. It has grown out of a desire to find a way for my informants to have a voice within the dissemination of my research. This approach is in line with reflexive and feminist approaches towards ethnography and applied anthropology. The chapter begins with the interlinked voices of two founding members of Zdravo Da Ste, Vesna Ognjenovic and Bojana Skorc, who are both also psychologists and academics. They outline the context of the work of Zdravo Da Ste and summarize their approach. This is followed by a summary of the methodological approach to my research, specifically focusing on my relationship to the field. In the next section, Vesna and Bojana give two examples of Zdravo Da Ste's work with children, which focus on play and the use of story respectively, and then discuss their work in relation to these examples. I follow this with a discussion of the use of play, creativity, story and the notion of 'meaning' in relation to my experience in the field and within a therapeutic perspective.

Approaches

Zdravo Da Ste – context and approach

In 1993 with the beginning of the civil war in former Yugoslavia, a group of psychologists were faced with a situation in which the psychology they had been taught could not be applied to the situation they were facing. Serbia hosted about one million refugee and IDPs from the war in former Yugoslavia, most of who did not repatriate. This was the biggest refugee crisis in Europe since the Second World War. According to the Serbian Commission for Refugees (SCR) after the biggest refugee crisis, operation 'Storm' in Croatia, the total number of officially recognized collective centres for refugees in Serbia was 700 (Serbian Commissariat for Refugees 2008). This was in addition to the unknown number of unofficial refugee centres, namely funded by private donations or in abandoned buildings. In 1999, following the new wave of refugee and IDP people and the Kosovo crisis, 388 new collective centres operated (Serbian Commissariat for Refugees 2008). Between 2000 and 2015 most of the newcomers were integrated into the local community and the number of refugees and IDPs decreased. Now in 2015, most of the refugees and IDPs have been integrated into the local community and have obtained Serbian citizenship. Collective centres are closing and few are now active. The people who still live in the collective centres are typically families with many children, and unemployed parents who have not had the opportunity to leave the collective centres and take responsivity for their families. They are socially marginalized. The office of the United Nations High Commission for Refugees (UNHCR) is still active, as well as SCR, but most of the people with whom they work now have citizenship.

Collective centres were the places in which refugee and IDP families were placed on arrival and the spaces within which they tried to re-establish their everyday lives. Most of the centres were inadequate for living, and had minimal hygiene facilities and limited personal space. Typically, one big space was divided into many smaller rooms in which family members lived and slept together. From a humanitarian point of view the situation within the collective centres was a very bad situation; however, from a psychological point of view this situation had hidden positive potentials alongside the negative. Children experienced collective life, and their families were extended to all people around them. In such situations, in many cases, family tragedy became part of a collective experience. Families were open to community more than was usual and got a chance to share their feelings, problems and hopes with other people. The group capacity to cope with crisis and develop strategies for overcoming them was bigger than any individual power.

It appeared to members of Zdravo Da Ste that the methodology that had been developed by individual psychology and clinical psychology, what they considered to be the most relevant parts of psychological education, was an insufficient response to the collective disaster. Many professionals were focusing on individual counselling, especially in work with women and children. The Zdravo Da Ste team noticed that new, more efficient and more general approaches were required in order to respond to the crisis. Individual approaches did not work because the general crisis and disaster were not situations for individual work. The streets were full of people, buildings were instantly transformed into refugee centres, and we were faced with large numbers of people and disorganized groups of children. Members of Zdravo Da Ste felt that an individual approach was required for a clear situation in which a minority of affected people were asking for help; the majority were not affected. This was a different situation from the one in which we found ourselves. Through our research we concluded that a dynamic and open social field was crucial for children's wellbeing and mental health (Ognjenovic, Andjelkovic & Skorc 1996). The basic ideas for a new approach were developed through practice and direct encounter with the people who were in need. This included a multidisciplinary approach, in which people are treated as active participants, co-creators of social events in a community context. The Zdravo Da Ste approach tended to introduce collective creativity, energy, wisdom and power in coping with personal tragedy.

The theoretical framework for Zdravo Da Ste's method was based on the social theory of Russian developmental psychologist Lev Vygotsky, specifically his theory of language and thought and the notion of the zone for proximal development (Vygotsky 1962). His basic idea was that psychological functions such as language, thought, speech and exploration are socially induced and have their origin in interaction between the child and its social partners – parents, siblings, friends, family. This suggests that the interactive field in which the child grows has the strongest and ultimate influence on development (Vygotsky 1981 [1960]). There is a dialectical relation between thought and activity in which practical exploration of thought creates new thoughts; this is how our experience is organized: 'Culture and development are related. Culture in a broadest sense. Personal development in a broadest sense' (Ognjenovic 2015). Zdravo Da Ste applied Vygotsky's ideas and developed key tenets.

They considered human development to be a process that lasts through the whole life. All participants within this process are partners in common activities, regardless of age, gender, ethnic, psychological or social status. The basic source of development is in building relations among people through conversations, expressions, new ways of playing and new activities – building relations among people through culture. Due to the lack of material supplies and basic security it appeared that social support and exchange were the strongest counter-balancing force that could give children and adults the chance to show and develop their human potentials. In accordance with Vygotsky's ideas idea Zdravo Da Ste developed social, interactive activities with children and their families.

A general framework for a programme of activities was developed in order to build activities aimed at supporting and promoting development. These were processes, not output-orientated. The programmes respected changes in a real-life context; they could not be fully defined in advance. The projects respected difference in its broadest sense. The focus was not on the unique but on mutual interactive benefits of human exchange. The patterns of interaction treated difference as a genuine social treasure out of which new ideas for new activities could be created.

Psychologists undertook the first steps in the development of Zdravo Da Ste's new approach, but it became clear that collective disaster and social crisis required a more complex approach. Artists, social workers, teachers and other professionals soon joined the Zdravo Da Ste team and became active creators of the approach. This was a new, creative possibility to open a process of building methodology. Method was not seen as a fixed form of activities and interventions, but as a chance to be constantly involved in the processes of restructuring it. The process was central and was, at the same time, the aim and the impact of the work. Participation in the activity was the goal for itself and through this process other new processes were initiated. The activities with children were not evaluated exclusively according to their effects, but also according to the whole complexity of the processes within and out of the children's life space. Understanding interaction as a process, involvement and activity are fundamental for creation not only of personal identity but the entire life experience.

The workshops for children were not created by adults; they were created through the common activities of adults and children through the relations between children and adults. The flexible structure of the workshops was open, creating possibilities and allowing transformation and integration into 'out-of-workshop' life events. They created the possibility of potential for development through interaction to become visible. Through the common activities of children and adults in a workshop context a mutual reconstruction of play and building relations with culture occurred. Play was the source of development.

In 2015 Zdravo Da Ste still have activities with children in three collective centres, and are in contact with many other people who are not in collective centres any more. Their professional network is available but is not active, as there are no funds. Members of Zdravo Da Ste work as volunteers. For the last two years they have received no support from Serbian institutions; they survive with the help of a Japanese donor. Zdravo Da Ste's method of working with children was related to a scientific theoretical frame, but is always partly independent. However strong the theory, it is the application that always adds value, overcoming basic ideas. The very process of application is at the same time a process of verification and modification. An efficient method is always rooted in life practice and must stay sensitive to relevant aspects of it. In this way, Zravo Da Ste's approach was and is continually developing and changing.

My methodology

I entered the field as a Dance Ethnographer but I participated in Zdravo Da Ste's workshops with children as both a Dance Ethnographer and DMP clinician engaging with the workshop participants through the different artistic media and activities in the workshops. The primary medium of communication between the children and myself were the activities themselves and the arts media used within the activities. As a member of the children's team and the Belgrade team, I contributed to the preparation and evaluation of the workshops in which I participated. In my fieldnotes I considered how the children had responded to the different media and how the workshops could be developed in response to the children's engagement with the artistic media and activities. Zdravo Da Ste introduced me to people in the field, as both a guest and a member of the Belgrade team. This gave me status, a role and responsibility, although this last aspect was of a lower degree than for other members of Zdravo Da Ste. Through this participation, I became an informal apprentice of Zdravo Da Ste. After several months of participation, I was given opportunities to co-facilitate workshops on their behalf. I also facilitated six practical presentations on different aspects of DMP for professionals working in the field.

As I began to understand Zdravo Da Ste's approach within their workshops with children and was increasingly given more practical responsibility within the activities, I was told I was no longer a guest but a member of the team who was asked and given permission to facilitate workshops with the children.

This was an important turning point, as it allowed me to apply my DMP skills more directly with the children. It also indicated that I was beginning to understand Zdravo Da Ste's approach, and therefore I could be trusted to co-facilitate and lead workshops on their behalf. My practical work in the field was thus an integration of my understanding of Zdravo Da Ste's approach and Dance Ethnography and DMP.

My integration of Dance Ethnography and DMP can be considered alongside applied anthropology (Chambers 1989; Ervin 2000; Kedia & Van Willigan 2005; Van Willigen 2002) and the application of ethnographic methods within the context of development studies (Arce & Long 2000a, 2000b). Applied anthropology can be understood as the use of anthropological skills and knowledge as a form of practical intervention (Van Willigen 2002). Anthropologist John Van Willigen (2002: 5–6) notes that one of a number of potential 'practitioner roles in anthropology' is the therapist, although he suggests this role is unusual (ibid). An applied anthropologist whose practitioner role is as a therapist uses his or her anthropological skills and knowledge alongside their therapeutic skills and knowledge in order to treat clients. In my research, although I integrated my anthropological and therapeutic skills, my aim was not to treat clients but to examine the use and meaning of movement and dance within Zdravo Da Ste's approach to psychosocial work with war-affected refugee people and IDPs. This is in line with an approach drawn from Dance Anthropology.

Dance anthropologists are concerned with understanding a particular group of people through comprehension of the dance systems they use. From the perspective of Dance Anthropology, dance can be perceived as 'structured movement systems . . . [socially constructed] systems of knowledge' (Kaeppler 1999:16), which give insight into the values and structures within a particular society. A contemporary approach towards Dance Anthropology, views dance as a form of human action (Hughes-Freeland 1999; Williams 1991). Dance anthropology utilizes ethnography as the primary method, where ethnography is both the process of gathering data, using participant observation, and the final written document, which constitutes the analysis of this data. Using ethnographic methods the dance researcher aims to understand the perspectives of the people in the field with respect to the meanings they give to movement and the context within which it is surrounded (Cowan 1990; Ness 1992; Sklar 2001). This is a classical approach to ethnography based on the ideas of anthropologist Bronislaw Malinowski (1992 [1922]). The completed ethnography can be seen as a way to understand the experience in the field so that the experience becomes integrated. It is a form of narrativization, and leads to new frames of meaning.

A central aspect of classical ethnography is participant observation. This can be considered more of a 'research strategy than a unitary research method' (Aull Davies 1999: 67) because it intrinsically employs many methods including formal and informal interviews, fieldnotes and journals, visual documentation and life histories. Anthropologist Charlotte Aull Davies (1999: 71) suggests that participation is important because it facilitates access to the field and possibilities for observation, which in turn highlight questions to be asked and areas to be understood. In participant observation, the researcher participates in the lives of the people being studied over an extended period of time, traditionally at least one year, in order to attempt to understand their perspectives of their lives and activities. This is called fieldwork. The researcher attempts to gain both an insider's and an outsider's perspective within the context of the field. As the fieldwork progresses, the ethnographer begins to move from being an outsider towards being an insider as they become more familiar with the different languages and texts of the field including embodied experience. Dance anthropologist Georgiana Gore suggests, 'Social acceptance as marked through dance indicates that one has found one's place in the other's world, a socio-spatial reorientation constructed in danced dialogue over time between Dance Ethnographer and other' (1999: 217). My fieldwork with Zdravo Da Ste took place over one year. I participated in Zdravo Da Ste's workshops with children and their families and attended meetings in preparation for these workshops. I undertook formal and informal interviews, kept fieldnotes and journals and used photography and video as media of documentation and participation. I took classes in the Serbian written and spoken language at a well-respected language school; and began to learn about the etno dance and the music of former Yugoslavia. I lived with a Serbian family and joined their personal and cultural celebrations. My participation in Zdravo Da Ste's workshops with children allowed me to begin to understand their approach to their work in an embodied sense and created a 'danced dialogue' through which I gained acceptance.

Sociologist Amanda Coffey (1999: 59) suggests fieldwork is an embodied activity in which the ethnographer is 'an embodied social actor' while the body itself serves 'as an agent of cultural reproduction and as a site of cultural representation' (ibid: 64). Embodied experience can thus be considered as a vehicle through which social norms and values can be learned, and culture represented. The embodied aspect of ethnographic research facilitates reflexivity as the researcher has the opportunity to become aware of their physical and emotional relationship to the field. It allows the researcher to distinguish between the meaning they may be imposing on a situation and the meaning given to the situation by the informants. Contemporary ethnography, in its application of 'ethnographic reflexivity' (MacDonald 2001: 68), allows a negotiation of meanings and understandings between the researcher and members of the field and considers both the people studied and the researcher as creators of meaning. This negotiation is acknowledged at all stages of the research. Dance anthropologist Theresa Buckland (1999: 7) suggests that reflexivity allows the power relations within the field and accompanying values and ethics to be exposed, particularly the often unequal relationship between the researcher and his or her informants.

In attempting to re-balance the power relations within the ethnographic process and adopt a collaborative approach to ethnography, my methodology moved towards a feminist ethnographic approach (Hopkins 1993). A feminist approach towards ethnography questions ethnographic representation, the ethnographic voice and views the researcher as 'a person with a distinct biography' (Hastrup 2004: 119). Anthropologist Sally McBeth (1993: 146–147) suggests there are both links and distinctions between a feminist and postmodern approach to anthropology in their concern with the role and voice of the researcher in relation to the subjects in the field. Similarly, my research and the work of Zdravo Da Ste have both integrated and negotiated the intertwining of diverse theoretical perspectives and methodologies. As Hastrup states, 'Ethnographies are realities, and their very incongruity reminds us about the plurality and generosity of the world' (Hastrup 2004: 129). Ethnographies reflect the reality of both the researcher and the fields in which they work. Part of my reality as an ethnographic researcher was that I was also a Dance Movement Psychotherapist.

DMP can be loosely defined as 'the use of creative movement and dance in a therapeutic relationship' (Payne 1992: 4). The client uses dance and movement within this relationship as media to facilitate change. Drawing on ideas from psychology DMP adopts the premise that 'it is the client, for whom the meaning has relevance in the personal situation, who, together with the therapist gives meaning to the work' (Payne 1992a: 6–7). The therapist may make connections, however, when reflecting on the session or through his or her movement observations in order to analyse and respond to movement created or presented by the client. DMP may incorporate other media, including visual images, music, voice, song and storytelling.

Within DMP there are a number of assumptions that form the foundations for theoretical principles. DMP presupposes, for example, that the mind and body mutually affect one another and are interlinked, so that a change in movement results in a change in the whole person (Payne 1992a, 1993a; Bernstein 1979; Schoop 1974; Meekums 2002). Through movement improvisation an individual can explore 'new ways of being' (Meekums 2002: 8). Play is also an important part of this process. Dance and movement are considered to be media of communication and expression and are assumed to have a symbolic function, which allows them to be representative of unconscious processes (Meekums 2002; Chaiklin & Schmais 1979; Chaiklin 1975; Payne 1992b; Stanton-Jones 1992). The individual is considered as having 'an innate capacity for continuous growth' (Bernstein 1979: 171–4) facilitated through the therapeutic relationship and process and mediated through both movement and words. The therapist also acknowledges his or her own embodied experience in relation to the therapeutic relationship, and this can provide insight. In DMP the notion of embodiment is concerned with the relationship between the individual's conception of themselves and the presentation of this self to others. DMP enables the client to explore these relationships and their use of the body as a form of representation and communication. The supervision process in DMP considers the embodied responses of the client and the therapist and the interactions between the two, thus creating a possibility for reflexive and reflective practice. I had monthly face-to-face and telephone clinical supervision with an experienced UK DMP clinician before, during and after my time in the field. This was alongside regular communication with my academic supervisor.

A DMP clinician who undertakes research within the context of their clinical practice becomes a practitioner–researcher (Rowan 1993). As in reflexive ethnographic work, the research process is engaged with 'multiple realities informed by a belief that research and knowledge is personal, social and cultural in construction' (Payne 1993b: 4). I felt that by incorporating DMP within my methodology I could use this understanding in an analysis of my observations.

Zdravo da Ste's examples of their approach to work with children

Example one

In one collective centre, in a town called Smederevo just south of Belgrade, was a boy who showed poor intellectual achievement, was not involved in primary education and was excluded from his peer group. He was unable to talk and could not participate in group play. After one year of participating in the Zdravo Da Ste programme, he started to speak in simple but expressive words, and to participate in and enjoy group activities. After three years of participating in the Zdravo Da Ste programme, he became accepted by the group and was able to participate in all activities. He is now respected as a person who can take care of younger participants and is sensitive to their needs. He is somebody who is different but is 'one of us'. The method of creative group activities gave him and his social field the chance to recognize and develop social skills that would not have been visible by other methods; especially not by the dominant education methods prevalent in Serbia at the time, which exclusively focused on intellectual development.

Example two

This is an example from a children's workshop held in March 1993, in which a play was created and performed by children from a collective centre in Belgrade.

Play: Let the Roses Flourish
Duration: 17 minutes
Place: Collective Centre Pionirski Grad in Belgrade

Actors: 5 refugee girls aged 5 to 9 in roles of adults, a child and roses.
Two girls played the parts of adults, the youngest girl was the child and four girls took the roles of roses.

Audience: A group of sixty people (refugee children and their families, other adults, elderly people, extended team of Zdravo Da Ste)

The male's destructive behaviour always made the roses fall down. Whenever roses fell down, the female started to raise them up by singing Flourish Roses. Her voice was gentle and her approaching movements gracious and protective. The roses responded consistently by rising up in slow motion. The roses were highly responsive to the interactions between adults, and reacted consistently to the male destructive behaviour and to female protective patterns. The episode of falling down and rising up was replicated sixteen times in the seventeen-minute play. They never got up by themselves and when they reached the upright position they could not retain it on their own. It was obvious that they needed constant support. They fell whenever the male approached, but they never manifested an active resistance to his severe attacks. They lay on the ground; they did not move or try to escape but responded consistently and promptly to the supporting efforts of the females.

Zdravo Da Ste's consideration of these examples

In the second example given above, the play was not fully prepared in advance. Only the initial phase of the play was structured: the main idea was globally defined and roles were divided up. The play was a fluid process, created jointly through acting. The male, female and child roles were recognizable through the play. The roles of roses was the original and joint creation of the children. This play was and still is relevant, and a prospective indicator of future developments because the children did something that was beyond them. To put this in developmental psychologist Lois Holzman's[2] words in reference to children's play:

> [T]he children are not acting but performing – creating new roles for themselves, reorganizing environmental scenes. In this sense, zpd (zone of proximal development) is a history game – the putting together of elements of the social environment in ways which help to see and show meaning-making as creative, productive activity.
>
> (Holzman, L 1997:73)

Many studies show that in an educational context as well as in everyday experiences there is not enough space for creativity and the building of new activities (Amabile 1996; Sternberg *et al.* 2005). Social situations and social tools such as personal names, self-portraits, the way we address others, the way we move, things we like or dislike, our personal spaces, expectations and the relations we build, all of these became tools for play activities within Zdravo Da Ste's workshops. Doing something with things that we would never usually do, telling things we never usually tell, being who we are not, drawing sounds, colouring thoughts or emotions, are all examples of some of the games we used, drawn from a list that is open-ended. The storytelling, drawing, creating associations to given creative material were effective in fostering creativity. They were associated with elaborated role-play and were nested in the developmental level of children's ability to improvise, pretend, perform, sing or dance. Vygotsky describes the activity of play as an explorative activity in which the child in cooperation with a social partner – other persons, playmates, parents as well as toys and cultural artefacts that contain interactive potentials – performs more than they could alone (Vygotsky 1962). In short, through interaction and play Zdravo Da Ste suggested that people actualize not only what they are but also what they are becoming and will potentially become in the future. This dynamic position is obtainable through play.

Faced with social crisis and collective disaster, it appeared that play activities were of crucial importance for psychological development and the creation of new identity. Play activity was seen as fundamental for child development. The child's capacity to play appeared to be an indicator of his or her psychological status and mental health. During the war, some children were exposed to extremely frustrating experiences. In the beginning, those children were not able to join the play; they lost the motivation and capacity to play and could not participate in activities with other children. They tended to withdraw, to be physically present but not absorbed by the activity of play. It was visible from their facial expressions and overall behaviour that they were not rejecting play but they were not able to play; they had lost the energy to play. We named this situation 'frozen play', and understood it as a reaction to negative experience.

In order to re-establish the capacity for play, the teams developed a non-invasive, step-by-step procedure. It became obvious that there was some order of play and expressive activities according to their applicability. If children lost their capacity to play, they could start with drawing. Children are typically not able to verbalize their feelings and experiences; they cannot talk about them even if their faces, bodies and whole appearance tell the story. Individual drawing without words is the first step to re-establishing play. It happened individually in the beginning, and after that the children were invited to join the group. Individual creative products were used for the next play activity. In the next step, we asked the children what we could all do with the drawings, not what they represented, and many of them gave suggestions. Suggestions were discussed, evaluated, accepted and practised with participation of all. In this way, the individual creative products became new tools for play and the children became involved in the play activity first, indirectly, through their remote contribution (drawing, word, written text, verbal reaction) and then directly, by active participation. Studies indicated that this methodology of social involvement in play activity significantly changes personal social capacities. In Zdravo Da Ste's approach, the individual and the group are not seen in opposition, but as interrelated forces, which results in common impact. In many of the dominant theories, the psychology of creativity treats the creative process as an individual process. The group is often seen as the background for individual achievement. The goal of the group leader is to set up a situation that can allow the individual to show his or her gift (Amabile 1996; Sternberg 1999; Sternberg *et al.* 2005). Some researchers have demonstrated the negative effects of group work on individual creativity (Kaufman & Sternberg 2010; Paulus Nijstad 2003). In many empirical approaches, the measure of group success is expressed as the sum of individual achievements. Evidently, there is a dominant assumption that the group influence is inter-individual, not intra-individual. This creates what can be described as a conceptual opposition between the two concepts. Recent authors, who implement the ideas of Vygostky, are overcoming this conceptual problem by seeing the relationship between the individual and group as a dynamic unit in which the individual is created by the group (Sawyer 2003; Sawyer *et al.* 2003). Zdravo Da Ste's workshop activities were focused on the group, seeing it as a dynamic field in which individual and group processes are interrelated. Group energy and group creativity became the sources for personal transformation. Participating in a group, a young person can express his or her feelings, fears, motives, expectations and at the same time participate in group feeling and creation. This is a two-way process, in which a person, at the same time, creates her or his identity on cultural, social and psychological levels. Zddavo Da Ste's workshops and activities were designed to allow interrelated development of individual and group expression.

In order to summarize our professional and human experience concerning the children affected by the war, we wish to make two points. First, the children's play-like activity is a condensed but not impoverished story about their lives. This has a prospective value under the war circumstances, because adult-initiated activity is reduced and impoverished. Second the children's persistence in growing and their need for the continual support of adults indicates a strong pro-life orientation. In this play, children became as if they were high above adults.

My understanding of Zdravo Da Ste's use of play and story

Within Zdravo Da Ste's work it appeared to me that relationships with play, creativity, story and other arts media were incorporated within the overall processes of the workshops. In this way seeds, rooted in metaphor, were planted which individual children might have the opportunity to explore further in their lives in the future. This reflected Zdravo Da Ste's intentions to integrate the workshop experiences within the everyday life of the participants and to allow the processes to continue and develop outside the workshop context.

Anthropologist Gregory Bateson identifies a relationship between the phenomenon of play and the process of therapy in terms of space and time. He suggests both use 'spatial and temporal bounding of a set of interactive messages. In both play and therapy, the messages have a special and peculiar relationship to a more concrete or basic reality' (2000: 191). Like the therapeutic space and Zdravo Da Ste's workshop space, the play space is set apart from everyday reality in space and time. Objects, relationships and activities take on a symbolic meaning not necessarily present in the everyday context. Within Zdravo Da Ste's workshops and within the play in an individual workshop, a separate time and space are created that is bounded spatially, emotionally and through the structure of the activities and the facilitators of the workshops. In this way a 'psychological frame' (Bateson 2000: 191) and a safe space is created in which the children and adults can explore relationships, emotions and questions.

Psychoanalyst D. W. Winnicott (1982) suggests play and creativity are directly related to the extent that it is only through play that a child or adult can 'be creative and . . . use the whole personality . . . it is only in being creative that the individual discovers the self' (Winnicott 1982: 63). Recognizing the ability to create allows the individual to harness and apply the resources inside themselves; and 're-arm' (Luria and Vygotsky 1992: 110–111). Vesna defined creativity in the following way 'I see creativity as life, it's not a means, it's not a tool, it's life and the people have . . . [an] endless capacity to create . . . To create means to be alive' (Ognjenovic 2001). Within the process of creativity something new is given form, recognized and put into relation with other things; in this way meaning and value are given. I feel this is the basis of DMP and Dramatherapy practice.

Members of Zdravo Da Ste talked to me more about creativity than they did about individual artistic media. When informants did talk to me about an individual 'medium, it was usually in the context of its being one of many creative elements that were applied in the workshops as part of a social frame . . . [or] social happening' (Tisma 2002), as illustrated in the story example given by Zdravo Da Ste earlier in this chapter.

Drama and play therapist Ann Cattanach (2002a: 191) suggests that stories have significance because they are socially and culturally situated and their meaning is negotiated between the listener, participants in the enactment of the story, and the teller. Through work with story and exploration of characters and situations within stories, participants have an opportunity to explore and recognize aspects of themselves and situations within their lives. Within Dramatherapy these aspects can be further explored through dialogues with clients, the development of roles identified within the stories, and the introduction of new tales. Story, and roles within the stories, are one of a number of vehicles that can facilitate the therapeutic process and interaction with metaphor (Jennings 1998; Gersie and King 1990; Jones 1996; Cattanach 2002a).

Child psychologist Bruno Bettleheim suggests that by identifying with a character, a child can 'compensate in fantasy and through identification for all the inadequacies, real or imagined' (1989: 57). The story and characters in a story become a metaphor for lived experience and present alternative possibilities in current or past experience. In order to make a story their own Bettleheim suggests a child needs to hear the story many times so that they can find what it has to offer them. I suggest that through familiarity with a story and by engaging and enacting characters from a story, a child has the possibility to embody those characters and through this process find new meaning and possibilities in relation to life experiences. This process of embodiment is important within the use of stories in a therapeutic context. It also highlights the way in which individual arts media are not necessarily divorced from one another.

Play therapist David Le Vay suggests that children have a 'narrative identity' which they 'carry within them' (2002: 36) as a way of understanding their experiences and the world in which they live. The personal and collective stories and other arts media created in Zdravo Da Ste's workshops can be seen as symbols placed in 'another social frame, not how it was, but how it is now' (ibid). The stories and other arts media thus created opportunities for the children to build new social and cultural relationships and place their experience within a different context. In this way the workshop process also allowed meaning to be found.

Bettleheim (1989 [1975]) suggests that the most important aspect of raising a child is to help them to find meaning in their lives. In the context of war-affected refugee and IDP people it is often necessary to find new frames of meaning as Art Therapists Debra Kalmanowitz and Bobby Lloyd (2005a: 24) found in their work with survivors of political violence in the UK and in Bosnia. I suggest that, by integrating different arts media within their aims and objectives, Zdravo Da Ste facilitated the development of new frames of meaning for the children and their families through verbal, non-verbal, embodied and tangible representations of experiences. Through these media and forms – play, story, dance and movement, visual imagery, etno, ritual and performance – participants had the opportunity to begin to understand and redefine themselves and their relationship to other people, and the social and physical environments by which they were surrounded. They could explore meaning in relation to their experiences of war and displacement and in this way create new physical, social and cultural relationships.

Conclusions

This chapter has attempted to present two voices from the field, that of two founding members of Zdravo Da Ste who are also psychologists, and that of myself as a Dance Ethnographer and Arts Psychotherapist. The social and methodological context of the research has been discussed; and the content, meaning and possible developmental implications of the activities of Zdravo Da Ste's workshops have been explored from both perspectives. This chapter reflects my attempt to create a piece of reflexive ethnography in which the different voices and meanings within the field can be heard and represented.

Although the methodology I adopted was effective in that it enabled me to gain access to the field and to interact with members of Zdravo Da Ste and the people with whom they worked, it was also problematic. My whole process of fieldwork was intertwined with Zdravo Da Ste's methods and approaches. Vesna suggested 'The differences among your work and our work are good, there is a dissonance but it is a good dissonance, it's not confrontational so that we can integrate and build new activities together' (Ognjenovic 2001). The most important difference was that Zdravo Da Ste did not consider their work to be therapy; they felt therapy was a closed and therefore limited form. Vesna also had two other concerns, first how my completed ethnography would be used by readers after it was completed; and second that she did not want me to represent Zdravo Da Ste in a public arena, since they could and did represent themselves. I carried these concerns and responsibilities with me throughout the research process.

In the context of the workshops I felt I had to put aside my preconceived notions of therapy in order to participate in the workshops. In the field I sometimes felt torn between my different roles and responsibilities; and questioned my task as a researcher and what it had to contribute to the profound and complex human situations in which I was participating and observing. In retrospect, the conflict that I experienced between the two methodologies actually served to further the research, in that it opened doors to new per-spectives and understanding. Moving between my role as Dance Ethnographer and Dance Movement Psychotherapist allowed me to gain inside knowledge of the field. Sociologists Alberto Arce and Norman Long suggest that an important aim of ethnographic studies within the context of international development is:

> to capture how people experience the establishment of new and the transformation of old codes of communication and to understand how they re-order their myths, images and 'monsters' (i.e., their fears, as well as their hopes and expectations) in narratives and practices which are held together through partial relations.

> (2000b: 27)

My research was inherently concerned with the 'establishment of new and the transformation of old codes of communication' and the re-ordering of 'myths, images and monsters,' which culminated in the beginnings of a shift in focus in the final stages of my research to the examination of the relationship between identity, symbols of identity and frames of meaning and their manipulation by the instigators of war and by Zdravo Da Ste. The ideas outlined by Arce and Long above explain why it was useful for me to adopt an ethnographic and reflexive approach and highlight the central concerns of my research and its relation to the wider discourse of anthropological study in the area of international development.

Notes

1   Etno was a term used by my informants to describe regional dance, music, and craft forms, including embroidery and carpentry, considered as arts of the people of former Yugoslavia, or Yugoslav folk arts. The term was also used to designate folk arts from other countries and regions. Etno represents specific regions of former Yugoslavia, recognized through particular visual motifs, rhythms, costumes or dance forms.
2   Lois Holzman is a developmental psychologist who works with vulnerable groups in the USA. She implements Vygotsky's ideas within her work. She is the director of East Side Institute for Short Term and Group Therapy and is involved in the All Stars Talents Show programme for youth in risk, and many other projects.

Bibliography

Amabile, T. (1996), *Creativity in Context*, USA: Westview.
Arce, A. & Long, N. (eds.) (2000a), *Anthropology, Development and Modernities*, London and New York: Routledge.
Arce, A. & Long, N. (2000b), 'Reconfiguring Modernity and Development from an Anthropological Perspective', in Arce, A. & Long, N. (eds.) *Anthropology, Development and Modernities* (pp. 1–31), London and New York: Routledge.
Aull Davies, C. (1999), *Reflexive Ethnography – A Guide to Researching Selves and Others*, London and New York: Routledge.
Bateson, G. (2000) [1972], *Steps to an Ecology of Mind*, Chicago and London: University of Chicago.
Bernstein, P.L. (ed.) (1979), *Eight Theoretical Approaches in Dance-Movement Therapy*, Iowa: Kendall/Hunt.
Bettleheim, B. (1989) [1975], *The Uses of Enchantment – The Meaning and Importance of Fairy Tales*, New York: Vintage.
Buckland, T.J. (1999), 'Introduction: Reflecting on Dance Ethnography', in T. J. Buckland (ed.) *Dance in the Field: Theory, Methods and Issues in Dance Ethnography* (pp. 1–10), London: Macmillan.
Cattanach, A. (2002a), 'The Narrow Road to the Deep North: Tracking a Life', in A. Cattanach (ed.), *The Story So Far – Play Therapy Narratives* (pp. 187–208), London: Jessica Kingsley.
Cattanach, A. (ed.) (2002b), *The Story So Far – Play Therapy Narratives*, London: Jessica Kingsley.
Chaiklin, S. (1975), 'Dance Therapy', in *American Handbook of Psychiatry*, New York: Basic.

Chaiklin, S. & Schmais, C. (1979), 'The Chace Approach to Dance Therapy', in P.L. Bernstein (ed.), *Eight Theoretical Approaches in Dance-Movement Therapy* (pp. 15–30), Iowa: Kendall/Hunt.

Chambers, E.I. (1989), *Applied Anthropology: A Practical Guide*, Prospect Heights, IL: Waveland.

Coffey, A. (1999), *The Ethnographic Self – Fieldwork and the Representation of Identity*, London, Thousand Oaks and New Delhi: Sage.

Cowan, J.K. (1990), *Dance and the Body Politic in Northern Greece*, Princeton, New Jersey: Princeton University.

Gersie, A. & King, N. (1990), *Storymaking in Education and Therapy*, London: Jessica Kingsley.

Gore, G. (1999), 'Textual Fields: Representation in Dance Ethnography', in T. J. Buckland (ed.) *Dance in the Field: Theory, Methods and Issues in Dance Ethnography* (pp. 208–20), Houndmills, Basingstoke, Hampshire and London: Macmillan Press; New York: St. Martin's Press.

Hastrup, K. (2004), 'Writing Ethnography – State of the Art', in J. Okely and H. Callaway (eds.), *Anthropology and Autobiography* (pp. 116–33), Abingdon, Oxon: Routledge.

Holzman, L. (ed.) (1997), *Schools for Growth*, New Jersey: Laurence Erlbaum.

Hopkins, M. C. (1993), 'Is Anonymity Possible? Writing About Refugees in the United States', in C.B. Brettell (ed.) *When They Read What We Write – The Politics of Ethnography* (pp. 121–31), Westport, Connecticut and London: Bergin and Garvey.

Hughes-Freeland, F. (1999), 'Dance on Film – Strategy and Serendipity', in T.J. Buckland (ed.) *Dance in the Field: Theory, Methods and Issues in Dance Ethnography* (pp. 111–22), Houndmills, Basingstoke, Hampshire and London: Macmillan Press.

Jennings, S. (1998), *Introduction to Dramatherapy – Theatre and Healing – Ariadne's Ball of Thread*, London and Philadelphia: Jessica Kingsley.

Jones, P. (1996), *Drama as Therapy – Theatre as Living*, Hove and New York: Brunner-Routledge.

Kaeppler, A. (1999), 'The Mystique of Fieldwork', in T.J. Buckland (ed.), *Dance in the Field: Theory, Methods and Issues in Dance Ethnography* (pp. 13–25), Houndmills, Basingstoke, Hampshire and London: Macmillan.

Kalmanowitz, D. & Lloyd, B. (2005a), 'Art Therapy and Political Violence', in D. Kalmanowitz, D. & B. Lloyd (eds.), *Art Therapy and Political Violence – With Art, Without Illusion* (pp. 14–34), Hove, East Sussex: Routledge.

Kaufman, R. & Sternberg, R. (2010), *The Cambridge Handbook of Creativity*, Cambridge: Cambridge University.

Kedia, S. & Van Willigen, J. (eds.) (2005), *Applied Anthropology: Domains of Application*, Westport, Conn: Praeger.

Le Vay, D. (2002), 'The Self is a Telling: A Child's Tale of Alien Abduction', in A. Cattanach (ed.) *The Story So Far – Play Therapy and Narratives* (pp. 35–58), Philadelphia: Jessica Kingsley.

Luria, A.R. & Vygotsky, L.S. (1992) [1930], *Ape Primitive Man, and Child: Essays in the History of Behavior*, New York and London: Harvester Wheatsheaf

McBeth, S. (1993), 'Myths of Objectivity and the Collaborative Process in Life History Research', in C.B. Brettell (ed.) *When They Read What We Write – The Politics of Ethnography* (pp. 145–63), Westport, Connecticut; London: Bergin and Garvey.

MacDonald, S. (2001), 'British Social Anthropology', in P. Atkinson *et al.* (eds.) *Handbook of Ethnography* (pp. 60–79), London, Thousand Oaks and New Delhi: Sage.

Malinowski, B. (1992) [1922], *Argonauts of the Western Pacific – An Account of Native Enterprises and Adventure in the Archipelagos of Melanesian New Guinea*, Routledge and Kegan Paul.

Meekums, B. (2002), *Dance Movement Therapy*, London, Thousand Oaks and New Delhi: Sage.

Ness, S.A. (1992), *Body, Movement, and Culture – Kinaesthetic and Visual Symbolisms in a Philippine Community*, Philadephia, Pensylavania: University of Pennsylvania.

Ognjenovic, V. (2001), *Interview with V. Ognjenovic in November 2001*, Belgrade, Serbia, [Recording in possession of Author].

Ognjenovic, V. (2015), Personal Communication with Author via Email on 30th January 2015, London.

Ognjenovic, V., Andjelkovic, D. & Skorc, B. (1996), 'Self Expression of Refugee Children Involved in the Program of Psychological Workshops, The Influence of Recent Socio-Political Events on Fine Arts and on Patient's Art', in *The American Society of Psychopathology of Expression* (pp. 181–202), New York.

Ognjenovic, V., Skorc, B. & Savic, J. (2003), *Social Sources of Life: Rehabilitation in the Former Yugoslavia-The Psychological Impact of War Trauma on Civilians – an International Perspective* (pp. 171–8), Westport, Connecticut: Praeger.

Paulus, P.B. & Nijstad, B.A. (2003), *Group Creativity: Innovation through Collaboration*, Oxford and New York: Oxford University Press.

Payne, H. (1992a) 'Introduction', in H. Payne (ed.) *Dance, Movement Therapy: Theory and Practice* (pp. 1–17), London and New York: Routledge.

Payne, H (ed.) (1992b), *Dance, Movement Therapy: Theory and Practice*. London and New York: Routledge.

Payne, H. (ed.) (1993a), 'From Practitioner to Researcher – Research as a Learning Process', in H. Payne (ed.) *One River, Many Currents – Handbook of Inquiry in the Arts Therapies* (pp. 16–40), London: Jessica Kingsley.

Payne, H. (ed.) (1993b) *One River, Many Currents – Handbook of Inquiry in the Arts Therapies*, London and Bristol, Pennsylvania: Jessica Kingsley.

Rowan, J. (1993), 'Foreword', in H. Payne (ed.) *One River, Many Currents – Handbook of Inquiry in the Arts Therapies* (pp. ix-x), London, Bristol and Pennsylvania: Jessica Kingsley.

Sawyer, R.K., John-Steiner, V., Moran, S., Sternberg, R.J., Feldman, D.H., Nakamura, J. & Csikszentmilayi, M. (2003), *Group Creativity: Music, Theater, Collaboration*, Mahwah, New Jersey and London: Lawrence Erlbaum.

Sawyer, K., John Steiner, V. Moran, S., Sternberg, R., Feldman, D. Gardner, H., Nakamura, J. & Csikszentmihalyi, M., (2003), *Creativity and Development*, Oxford: Oxford University Press.

Schoop, T. (1974), *Won't You Join the Dance – A Dancer's Essay into the Treatment of Psychosis*, Palo Alto: National.

Serbian Commissariat for Refugees (2008), *Situation and Needs of Refugee Situation in The Republic of Serbia*. Available online at: www.kirs.gov.rs/docs/RefugeeNeeds AsessmentReportSerbia.pdf (accessed 27 July 2015).

Sklar, D. (2001), *Dancing with the Virgin – Body and Faith in the Fiesta of Tortugas, New Mexico*, Berkeley, Los Angeles and London: University of California.

Stanton-Jones, K. (1992), *An Introduction to Dance Movement Therapy in Psychiatry*, London: Routledge.

Sternberg, R. (1999), *Handbook of Creativity*, Cambridge: Cambridge University.

Sternberg, R., Grigorenko, E. & Singer, J. (2005), *Creativity – from Potential to Realization*, Washington, DC: American Psychological Association.

Tisma, B. (2002), *Interview with Branka Tisma in March 2002*, Belgrade, Serbia. [Recording in possession of Author].

Van Willigen, J. (2002), *Applied Anthropology: An Introduction* (3rd edn.), Westport, CO: Bergin and Garvey.

Vygotsky, L.S. (1962), *Thought and Language*, Cambridge, MA: MIT Press; New York: John Wiley & Sons.

Vygotsky, L.S. (1981) [1960], 'The genesis of higher mental functions', in J.V. Wertsch, (ed.) *The Concept of Activity in Soviet Psychology* (pp. 144–188), Armonk, NY: Sharpe.

Williams, D. (1991), *Ten Lectures on Theories of the Dance*, Metuchen, NJ and London: The Scarecrow.

Winnicott, D.W. (1982) [1971], *Playing and Reality*, Harmondsworth, Middlesex: Penguin.

Zdravo Da Ste (2006), *Zdravo Da Ste/Hi Neighbour*. Available online at: www.zdravodaste.org.rs (accessed 24 February 2006).

Chapter 9

Voice of the object

Art psychotherapy and translating cultures

Margaret Hills de Zárate

Introduction

In a world increasingly characterized by transnational and globalized connections, the need for understanding and communication within, between and across diverse cultures is stronger than ever. The Arts and Humanities Research Council 'Translating Cultures' research theme proposes that this need can be addressed by studying the role of translation, understood in its broadest sense to include the transmission, interpretation and sharing of languages, values, beliefs, histories, narratives and life stories, and the vehicles of translation, such as art, performances, objects and other cultural artefacts. 'Translation' is thus conceived as relating to processes that are not exclusively inter-lingual (between languages) but also those processes that are intermedial (between media) or inter-cultural (between cultures) and encompass issues such as the 'untranslatability', and the impact of what is transformed, gained or lost in the process of translation (Forsdick 2014). I propose that these processes have clear parallels to those at play in the practice of a culturally sensitive art psychotherapy informed by ethnographic and sociocultural perspectives.

Overview of research

My research is located in the 'Transnationalizing Modern Languages: Mobility, Identity and Translation in Modern Italian Cultures' research project, one of the three large grants under the overarching Translating Cultures theme. It involves researchers at four UK universities – Bristol, Warwick, St Andrews and Queen Margaret University – and a number of academic and community partners across the world, all engaged in the investigation of practices of linguistic and cultural interchange and the exploration of the ways in which cultural translation intersects with linguistic translation in our everyday lives. While this specific project focuses on the case of Italian mobility, identity and translation in modern Italian cultures, it is intended to provide a template from which to develop a new paradigm for the work of modern language studies and its applications in the twenty-first century through the close study of Italy's particular and complex history of migrations (Burdett 2014). The potential for this development will be through the generation of multiple case studies of Italian migration across the world, from Argentina to Ethiopia, which will contribute towards a larger category of research, in turn aimed at generating new understandings of cultural translation in all its multiple manifestations in the context of our rapidly changing, globalized world (Flyvbjerg 2006; Blommaert & Dong Jie 2010). The aims of this research theme are multiple and far reaching, with the exploration of key concepts such as multiculturalism, multilingualism, tolerance, intolerance and identity at its core. These concepts, and my specific focus on intermediality, which in this research involves and seeks to examine the relationship between the visual and the verbal and the movement from one representation to another, have implications for the practice of art psychotherapy.

My own work as a co-investigator in this research project focuses on transgenerational Italian migration in South America, taking four major sites as specific areas of study – Buenos Aires in Argentina, São Paulo in Brazil, Montevideo in Uruguay and Valparaiso in Chile. The methodology for my current research in the 'Transnationalizing Modern Languages' research project' has evolved from previous ethnographic research undertaken in Cuba, the Republic of Georgia, Colombia and Ukraine and involves a range of approaches to community participation in researching the lived experience of participants and involving them directly in the co-creation of the research. These participative approaches include workshops, focus groups and individual interviews. The examples referred to here are limited to fieldwork in Argentina.

Italians in Buenos Aires

The history of Italians and of Italian culture in Argentina has its roots in multiple experiences of mobility and transnationalism that can be traced back to the seventeenth century. However, the large-scale migration of Italians can be described as occurring in distinct waves: 1876–1895, mainly from the northern regions of Piedmont, Veneto and Lombardy; 1895–1914, when migration patterns shifted to rural and former independent Southern Italy, especially Campania, Calabria and Sicily; and finally a third wave, from 1946–1957, in the years following the end of the Second World War (Mignone 2008; Devoto 1984, 2006). As Schneider (2000) notes 'the massive movement of peoples in search of a better life in the nineteenth and early twentieth centuries was the product of specific internal factors of poor areas in Europe, which could not provide subsistence for their population and repressed demands for redistribution of wealth and the opportunities offered by the rising economies in the New World' (Schneider 2000: 61). Transatlantic networks informed Italians, of the economic opportunities in Argentina in both commercial and agricultural sectors of what was then a booming economy.

The great majority of Italian immigrants to Argentina arrived as poor, often illiterate, unskilled or semi-skilled workers, many of them peasants or agricultural workers. In general, Northern Italians went to rural Argentina whereas South Italians tended to go to cities, particularly Buenos Aires (Schneider 2000). In Buenos Aires, at the turn of the century, Italians joined the growing urban economy and found occupational niches such as tailors, and fruit and vegetable vendors, and contributed largely to the rise of manufacturing, mechanical, food processing, textile and furniture-making industries (Schneider 2000). An urban industrial elite developed, largely of Italian origin. It maintained strong links of patronage with the local Italian working class, its workforce and consumers, through the control of numerous mutual-aid associations (*società di mutuo soccorso* or *sociedades de socorros mutuos*) (Scarzanella 1981; Devoto 1984). I gained access to my respondents with the collaboration of these societies, whose membership was largely descended from the two main Italian populations Friuli Venezia and Calabria referred to in the literature. As most arriving immigrants spoke regional dialects of Italian, they found it easier to communicate in Spanish, which became their shared language.

Methodologies: ethnography and ethnographic and participatory approaches

The methodology for my current research in the 'Transnationalizing Modern Languages' research project evolved from previous ethnographic research undertaken in Cuba, the Republic of Georgia, Colombia and Ukraine.

Ethnography quite literally means to 'write' (or represent) a culture. It is not a specific data collection technique, but rather a multiple technique approach by which the ethnographer can adapt and draw upon a mix of methods appropriate to a situation. Research and data collection take the form of diverse experiences, workshops, encounters, relationships, observations, and conversations as opposed to closely structured interviews, as it is only as the conversations and interviews progress that the next question emerges (Parthasarathy 2008), an inductive approach not dissimilar to that adopted by the therapist as reflexive practitioner (Finlay 2008: 3). As Hoey (2014) points out 'an ethnography may be defined as both a qualitative research process or method (one conducts an ethnography) and product (the outcome of this process is an ethnography) whose aim is cultural interpretation' (Hoey 2014: 1). The ethnographer goes beyond reporting events and details of experience. Like the psychotherapist, the ethnographer attempts to understand how these events or reported experiences represent what Geertz (1973) has called 'webs of meaning', referring to the cultural constructions by which we live and the analysis of them. Ethnography, like psychotherapy, is therefore not an experimental science in search of law but an interpretative one in search of meaning (Hoey 2014; Seeley 2004, 1999). These 'webs of meaning' or 'significance' underlie society, human interactions including our thoughts and emotions, by 'providing a background set of assumptions and values that set restraints on human functioning and orientate us to what is meaningful' (Tsoi Hoshmand 2006: 188).

Our assumptions and values extend to material culture, which focuses on objects, their properties, the materials that they are made of, and the ways in which these materials are central to an understanding of culture and social relations (Woodward 2013) including the making of and relationship with images and artefacts. The cultural dimensions of material and visual cultures as represented in art-making through choices of materials, subject matter and the use of symbols and metaphor must, therefore, be considered in art psychotherapy practice (Bird 2012; Hogan 2015; Hogan and Pink 2011; Hocoy 2005; Hocoy 2002; Landes 2012) if art psychotherapists are to engage in any meaningful way with clients from backgrounds different from their own. Shweder's (1991) definition of the field of cultural psychology as 'the study of the ways subject and object, self and other, psyche and culture, person and context, figure and ground, practitioner and practice, live together, require each other, and dynamically, dialectically, and jointly make each other up' is helpful in outlining what this involves (Shweder 1991: 73). Moreover, it describes 'a non-reductionistic approach to understanding the interrelatedness of aspects in the human domain' of interest to psychotherapists, ethnographers and social scientists (Tsoi Hoshmand 2005: 2).

Fieldwork

Fieldwork is one of the key principles of ethnography whereby the eth-nographer spends extended periods of time in the everyday environment of a culture or group of individuals under study collecting data. However, as Blommaert and Dong Jie (2010) point out, this is true only to some extent for while one should, of course, 'return from the field loaded with bags full of "data": raw and half-processed materials that reflect and document the realities in the field . . . fieldwork should not just be reduced to data collection, because essentially it is a learning process' (Blommaert and Dong Jie 2010: 27). Apart from an initial period of prolonged fieldwork in Havana (Hills de Zárate 2010, 2011), most of my research has involved shorter periods of immersion, due to limited economic resources and work commitments (Hills de Zárate 2012). In such situations, I have used an ethnographic approach congruent with what Jeffrey and Troman (2004) describe as a 'compressed time mode', which involves a shorter period of intense ethnographic research in which 'researchers inhabit a research site almost permanently for anything from a few days to a few months, involve themselves in the life of the inhabitants, and seek access to as many site contexts and people as possible'. I have also employed a 'selective intermittent time mode', where the length of time spent doing research is longer but with a very flexible approach to the frequency of site visits (Jeffrey and Troman 2004: 538–40).

As a healthcare professional I was granted immediate entry to both the site and population and attached to a multidisciplinary team looking at the potential implementation of art therapy within existing psychosocial models of practice with refugees in such diverse settings as the Republic of Georgia, Colombia and Kenya. However, to be able to do this, it was essential to understand the context in which this could be achieved and also to identify what approach to art therapy might be beneficial, given the multiple issues at play such as safety, temporality, continuity, confidentiality and culture. Access to multiple gatekeepers in the multidisciplinary team in turn facilitated direct access to key members within the communities.

A gatekeeper is an individual who facilitates access to the site and to participant subjects. Such a role implies someone with authority or ownership in line with the existing cultural norms of the research setting, which in my case were mainly other healthcare professionals or aid organisations (Sanders 2006). However, as Christian (2012) notes 'depending on the place, nature and participant body of research subjects, the role of gatekeeper can be anything from one of simple formality to one of extraordinary complexity, where sought after access is deeply embedded into the research project such as when gatekeepers are also participants and subjects' (Christian 2012: 2).

Case vignette: are you a journalist?

One example of this involved working with a group of adolescent boys, one of whom occupied various roles in my research – key informant, gatekeeper and latterly co-researcher. As gatekeeper he introduced me to his family and other community members, and when I decided not to take photographs following a conversation with a local man about press coverage, which revealed that many journalists had visited the camp and that their presence had been experienced as intrusive and their reports inaccurate and misrepresentative, he took over the role and as a co-researcher the collection of visual material relating to this piece of work, providing an insight into the camp based on what he thought was important for others to be aware of and which might otherwise have remained invisible to me. As I did not know what I did not know, I had to rely on my respondent to show me (Lincoln & Guba 1985: 269). Ultimately, the researcher's ability to navigate through gatekeepers at many levels and of varying connectivity to the research-subject community is essential to any fieldwork success (Christian 2012). While I cannot claim to have 'planned' this particular interaction, such an approach is in keeping with participatory research methods that are geared towards 'planning and conducting the research process with those people whose life-world and meaningful actions are under study' (Bergold & Thomas 2012: 1).

This particular episode occurred during what Whitehead (2005) refers to as the 'initial ethnographic tour' of the research site in rural or small communities. Often conducted as walks, the ethnographer may begin 'unstructured or natural conversational interviews' with people encountered or a member of the community will engage the ethnographer in conversation. Through such processes the ethnographer 'may eventually identify participants for further semi-structured or even structured interviews, as well as meet additional community members' (Whitehead 2005: 16). Conversations such as the 'are you a journalist conversation' described would I think fit Whitehead's definition of a 'natural conversational ethnographic interview', as the discourse is similar to what naturally occurs in a conversation, and usually occurs when the ethnographer is simply another participant in a conversation, as indeed I was. However, as Whitehead (2005) goes on to point out, once in the field one is alert to material that pertains to the object of one's research.

> Ethnographers having some idea of what it is that they want to learn in the setting, aspects of their research concerns are never far from their consciousness, even though the conversation or the activity may be primarily social or informal. Because some form of research paradigm is part of an ethnographer's consciousness, she or he is not only alert when something emerges in the conversation in which they don't quite understand, but also when the conversation seems to be moving into an area related to that research paradigm.
>
> (Whitehead 2005: 16)

Having gained entry, in my case to Italian communities in Buenos Aires, the next step is to proceed to collect the material required in order to answer one's research questions. This requires a research methodology, and underpinning any methodology is a set of epistemological positions and values as expressed through the approaches I have adopted.

Participatory approaches to research

Participatory research can be regarded as a methodology that argues in favour of the possibility, the significance and the usefulness of involving research partners in the knowledge-production process (Bergold 2007). Participatory approaches are not fundamentally distinct from other empirical social research procedures; there are numerous links, especially to qualitative methodologies and methods. Participatory research involves collaborative research activities. Especially in health research, funders now recognize that the involvement of service users in the research process makes good sense. Public and patient involvement (PPI) in research is now explicitly required by most funding bodies (Cook 2012). Approaches that seek to close the gap between ethnography and community engagement include Community-based Ethnographic Participatory (CBEP) research, which focuses on culture and cultural interpretation and uses a participatory process undertaken with community members (Israel, Eng, Schulz & Parker 2013). However, CBEP is usually large scale, long term, and involves a team of researchers including both academic and community members (Parrado, McQuiston & Flippen 2005; Austin 2003; Lassiter 2000). My own experience is closer to that described by Cheney (2011), who used a participatory ethnography approach in a six-week period in the field involving young local people as research assistants in assessing orphans' needs in Africa and who states that 'the truth is that every research participant, every friend and cultural guide, is a collaborator in building our cultural interpretations' (Cheney 2011: 170). In developing my own ethnographic stance, I have found the voice of Barbara Tedlock (1991) reassuring:

> However the discipline (of ethnography) may develop historically, there currently exists a (new) breed of ethnographer who is passionately interested in the co-production of ethnographic knowledge, created and represented in the only way it can be, within an interactive Self/Other dialogue.
>
> (Tedlock 1991: 82)

In my current research, I have employed a 'selective intermittent time mode' (Jeffrey and Troman 2004) i.e. blocks of immersion in the field coupled with visits to the sites of emigration in Italy as a means of sensitizing myself to environments left behind or, in the case of transgenerational migration, imagined cultural landscapes. Contact with key respondents, who are invited to 'write into' transcriptions of interviews, has been maintained through the Internet. I have also focused on material culture and the world of objects as a medium of cultural translation.

Objects

The Transnationalizing Modern Languages research involves an examination of the role of objects in mediating constructions of identity in relation to transgenerational migration. One research question is how processes of translation occur within material culture, in particular, those processes that are intermedial. Intermedial (between media) refers to speaking about objects, or (at the risk of being fanciful) when the object speaks to us.

The relationship between people and objects has been the focus of material culture studies defined by Miller (1983) as an 'integrative' field, drawing across disciplines to examine 'a core relationship between objects and people' (Miller 1983: 5). The literature pertaining to this 'integrative field' emanates from a variety of sources including history, art history, art, psychology, psychoanalysis, sociology, anthropology and cultural studies, that is, the same range of disciplines that inform the discipline of art psychotherapy. One example is Miller's ethnographic study of a London street, a collection of thirty narrative portraits of individual homes, the people who live in them and their possessions. He argues that human relationships are central to modern life and that material culture is fundamental in underpinning these relationships. Miller's study focuses on people's relationships with material objects, which are viewed as 'an integral and inseparable aspect of all relationships' (Miller 2008: 286). The central thrust of his research is to 'challenge our common-sense opposition between the person and the thing, the animate and the inanimate, the subject and the object' (2010: 5).

In conducting his research, Miller asked people about the interiors of their homes, the decoration, the choices that had been made and the objects displayed. By enquiring about things, as opposed to more direct personal questions, he found that people shared a great deal more about themselves than they otherwise might have in a more traditional interview. One advantage of adopting this 'unusual perspective', (Miller 2010) but which should come as no surprise to art therapists, is that these apparently mute, inanimate forms often 'spoke' more easily and eloquently to the nature of relationships than people themselves. Another, but unexpected, outcome was that participants in the study often used the encounter as an occasion to re-examine and, to some degree, to re-evaluate their lives (Miller 2008: 296).

In defining objects as 'things' or 'stuff' Miller takes a view with which I sympathize, in that he refuses to offer a clear definition of what constitutes these objects, arguing that 'to try to determine the exact criteria by which some things would be excluded, as perhaps less tangible, or too transient, would be a hopeless exercise' (Miller 2010: 1). Between April and May 2015 I ran a series of workshops in Buenos Aires and Cordoba in Argentina entitled 'Objects, mementos and narratives: an exploration of transgenerational identity', which were advertised as follows:

> The specific objective of this workshop is the exploration of trans-generational identity as mediated by objects and our use of them. Objects, from photographs to the souvenir or memento, and the practices associated with them; function as vehicles that facilitate the expression of cultural identity. Participants are invited to bring a personal item, which represents their relationship, real or symbolic, with the concept of heritage and identity. The orientation workshop will be dynamic, practical and thematic although essentially non-directive. Participants should be prepared to participate in the experience of artistic creation and be willing to share and exchange their experiences with others.[1]

The objects that participants brought to these workshops were varied beyond any expectation. For the purposes of this chapter I will briefly discuss one workshop held in Morón, a town on the outskirts of Buenos Aires, where the following objects were brought:

> A tiny souvenir of a Sicilian horse and cart carefully repaired: a coffee grinder, a coffee pot, and a beautifully preserved dress that had once belonged to one participant's grandmother who had been a seamstress.

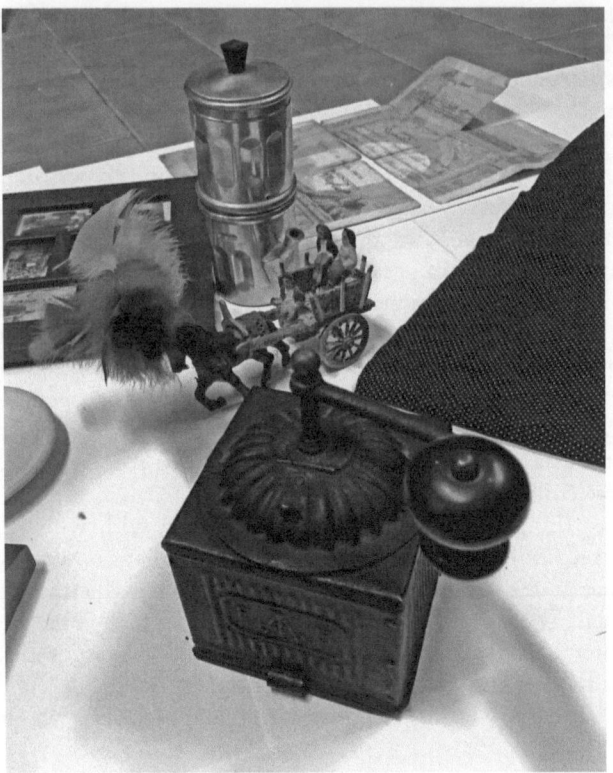

Figure 9.1 Objects, mementos and narratives: an exploration of transgenerational identity, *Societá Italiana di Mutuo Soccorso di Morón*, April 2015

Photographs, a photograph album from Japan, certificates, passports and a tiny plate.[2]

All of these objects corresponded, if not to a person, to a sense of identity. · One respondent who was willing (among many) to be interviewed about the connection between object and life history was interviewed following the workshop. An important culture bearer (Friedman 1994) was her grandfather Ruggerio Vannella, whose photograph she brought to the group. A gypsy from Mola di Bari and a musician, his granddaughter was training to be a medical doctor; she carries his name and a powerful sense of personal identity related to him and the objects left behind following his death. One thought that arose, and was reiterated in another interview with a retired doctor, was that these relationships of caring or witnessing caring had informed their choice to become doctors.

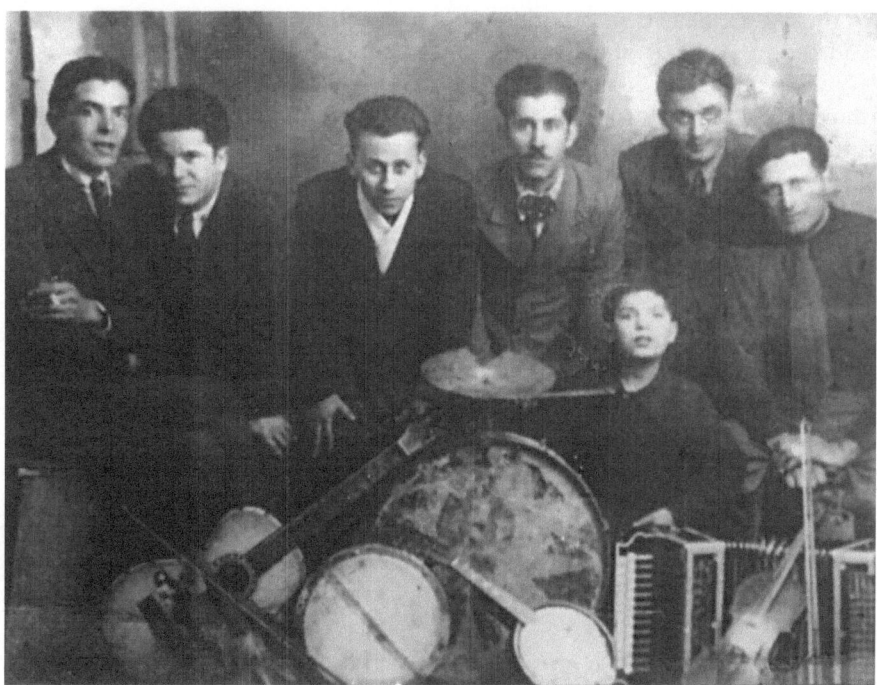

Figure 9.2 Ruggiero Vannella (far left) and the Orchestra Jazz Adriatica Sinfonica, Mola di Bari, Puglia, Italia

Intermediality

The link between the object and what it represents involves the translation of material culture to a narrative. In order to conceptualize this relationship, the concept of intermediality is needed. Intermediality is a way of understanding the relations between two (or more) media, such as writing, speech and images, or the transgression of boundaries between them. As previously noted, 'translation' is conceived as relating to processes that are not exclusively inter-lingual but also processes that are intermedial, between different media (Forsdick 2014), and these processes are at play in the workshop scenarios, such as the one previously described when we imbue our material world and the objects within it with narrative. However, these processes can be safely harnessed to explore other social phenomena beyond the clinical setting if the focus of the research is inductive, that is to say, if the researcher does not attempt to impose a priori interpretations on the material that surfaces. Examples of similar research include Miller (2005, 2008, 2010), as well as Turkle (2011) who has published a collection of autobiographical essays, on the evocative nature of things by scientists, humanists, artists, and designers trace the power of objects in their lives, objects that Turkle (2011) classifies according to the association and the meaning attributed to it by the author. Turkle (2011) invites us to consider objects as companions to our emotional lives or as provocations to thought, and presents us with objects of discipline and desire, objects of history and exchange, transition and passage, underscoring the inseparability of thought and feeling in our relationship to things.

Literature is replete with such explorations as in Proust, or Walter Benjamin's 'Berlin around 1900', the greater part of which was written when Benjamin lived in exile in Paris. Benjamin attempts to reconstruct his own past life, as well as the life of an epoch, as they were shaped by a city. Unpublished in his own lifetime, Benjamin uses the objects, interiors and experiences of his childhood to explore the relationship between people, memory and things. One object, the 'reading box', a box full of lettered tablets with which to form words, stands out, of which he writes:

> Everyone has encountered certain things which occasioned more lasting habits than other things. Through him or her, each person developed those capabilities, which helped to determine the course of his life . . . none of the things that surrounded me in my early years arouses greater longing than the reading box.
>
> (Benjamin 2006: 16)

Benjamin's account of the reading box describes longing for a lost world, but it is also a description of the beginning of a life of writing and, I think, an example of what Miller (2010) is referring to when he states that people not only make things, but things make people. By this, Miller is referring to the way in which we are unconsciously shaped by the things that surround us in an exterior environment that habituates and prompts us (Miller 2010: 51). In developing his theory of things, Miller acknowledges his debt to the French anthropologist and sociologist Pierre Bourdieu, who defines this exterior environment as 'habitus . . . a durable, transposable system of definitions' acquired initially by the young child as a result of the conscious and unconscious practices of her/his family (Bourdieu & Wacquant 1992: 126–7). Habitus is 'embodied history, internalised as second nature and so forgotten as history' (Bourdieu 1990: 56). In other words, habitus is historically conditioned and deeply internalized, thus forming a kind of second nature and giving our thoughts, feelings and actions their apparently 'natural', or 'spontaneous' character. The habitus is a generative rather than a fixed system: a basis from which endless improvisations can derive, a 'practical mastery' of skills, routines, aptitudes and assumptions that leave the individual free to make (albeit limited) choices in the encounter with new environments or fields. Written in exile from a world he could never return to, memory is conceived as a palimpsest in which Benjamin peels away the layers of history to expose the foundational traces of his early life, the reading box, and a return to the primary habitus (Sleight 2006).

Reflexivity

The degree of involvement that ethnography involves requires considerable flexibility and reflexivity. A reflexive approach in ethnography enables one to understand how the researcher who is also a practitioner has an impact on those researched. It also implies that the researcher with such a background should interrogate their own beliefs and feelings in the same way that they interrogate those of others (Arber 2005). This process has much in common with reflective practice and reflexive thinking, which are essential components of therapy as both the therapist and researcher become a part of the very process that they are trying to step back from and observe (Stedmon & Dallos 2009).

Stedmon and Dallos (2009) suggest that reflective practice in psychotherapy is best seen as a successive process of analysing and reanalysing important episodes of activity, drawing on multiple levels of representation including propositional, autobiographical and ethical knowledge and helpfully distinguishing personal reflection from personal reflexivity.

The term personal reflection is used to refer to the spontaneous and immediate act of reflecting in the moment, and is restricted to describing reflection in action, most usually during therapy, but also applied to other professional contexts such as supervision, consultation, teaching and learning. Personal reflection typically encompasses self-awareness of bodily sensations and emotions and the attentional focus on memories, experiences and cognitions as evoked during in-the-moment reflective episodes. In contrast, personal reflexivity refers to the act of looking back over, or reflecting on, action. This implies a meta-theorized processing of events retrospectively, where the original episode of reflection becomes the object of further conscious scrutiny. Personal reflexivity is primarily a conscious cognitive process whereby knowledge and theory are applied to make sense of remembered reflective episodes. This draws on multiple sources of prior knowledge, including model-specific theories of psychological processes, a theorized understanding of one's own social status and situation in terms of gender, class and ethnicity, and self-narratives that represent autobiographical accounts that story our own life experiences. Thus 'personal reflexivity' refers to 'the way that the [therapist or researcher] acknowledges how her own agendas, experiences, motivations and political stance contribute to what goes on in work with clients' (Stedmon & Dallos 2009).

Both personal reflection and reflexivity are involved in ethnography: the former in relation to being and doing in the field, and the latter in the learning and making sense of the material collected there. These are also elements of auto-ethnography.

Evocative or analytic auto-ethnography

Auto-ethnography is a qualitative research method that combines characteristics of ethnography and autobiography within the creative and performing arts as

a research tool (Pace 2012). However, while auto-ethnography is now established as a useful research method, it has also been criticized for its rejection of
traditional analytic goals such as abstraction and generalization (Anderson
2006a; Atkinson 2006). Ellis (2004) argues that autoethnographies do contain
analytic elements in the sense that 'when people tell stories, they employ analytic
techniques to interpret their worlds' (2004: 195–196). However, this form of
analysis does not sit comfortably with the realist or analytic tradition. On the
subject of generalization, Ellis argues that it is possible to generalize from an
auto-ethnography, but not in a traditional manner. 'The generalisability of an
auto-ethnography is tested by readers as they determine if the story speaks to
them about their experience or about the lives of others they know' (Ellis 2004:
194–195). The autoethnographer does not privilege traditional analysis and
generalization. Anderson (2006a) has expressed concerns about certain aspects
of the 'evocative or emotional' auto-ethnographic method championed by Ellis
and Bochner (2000) and other symbolic interactionists with postmodern or
poststructuralist sensitivities (Denzin 2006). Anderson (2006), while applauding
efforts in articulating and exemplifying this emergent research method, has also
expressed fear that 'evocative or emotional autoethnography' may have the
unintended consequence of eclipsing other visions of what auto-ethnography
can be and of obscuring the ways in which it may fit productively in other
traditions of social inquiry (Anderson 2006a: 374). Dissatisfied with the
limitations that evocative auto-ethnography places on researchers who want to
practise auto-ethnography within a realist or analytic tradition, he proposes an
alternative research method that is committed to an analytic agenda named
'analytic autoethnography' to distinguish it from the 'evocative or emotional
autoethnography' promoted by Ellis and Bochner (2000).

> The purpose of analytic ethnography is not simply to document personal
> experience, to provide an "insider's perspective," or to evoke emotional
> resonance with the reader. Rather, the defining characteristic of analytic
> social science is to use empirical data to gain insight into some broader set
> of social phenomena than those provided by the data themselves.
>
> (Anderson 2006: 386–87)

Ellis and Bochner (2006) and Denzin (2006) have opposed Anderson's
proposal on the grounds that it could dilute the current meaning of the term
'autoethnography'; it could contain, limit or silence the researcher's self in
the research context; and it could reduce publishing opportunities for those
who seek to practice evocative auto-ethnography. Other ethnographers, such
as Charmaz (2006) and Pace (2012), have welcomed it. In my own research,
I am currently looking at both models, but given that my work is part of
a contribution to a greater whole, that of the 'Transnationalizing Modern
Languages' project, veering towards Anderson's proposal to use grounded theory

at the stage of analysis of the data collected in diverse sites over the life of the project. Some art psychotherapists have used elements of auto-ethnography to great effect (Hocoy 2006; Schaverien 1998) in relation to a cultural identity.

Generalization

It is important to emphasize that the object of investigation in ethnography is always a uniquely situated reality: a complex of events, which occurs in a totally unique context – time, place, participants, even the weather. The ethnographer is always working in a series of conditions that can never be repeated. Even if events look or seem to be the same, they never are because they are different events happening at another time. This brings us to the issue of representativeness. What sort of relevance do these very specific snapshots of reality have and how confidently can generalizations be drawn from the data collected? The answer lies in the fact that ethnography is an inductive science, that is: it works from empirical evidence towards theory, not the other way around. You follow the data, and the data suggest particular theoretical issues (Bloommaert & Dong Jei 2010). This approach has clear parallels with the practice of art psychotherapy if we follow the information and material provided by the patient, which in turn suggests the therapeutic intervention. The discrete ethnography is presented, as a case study, which 'properly understood, is not simply the report of an event or incident. To call something a case is to make a theoretical claim – to argue that it is a 'case of something', or to argue that it is an instance of a larger class' (Shulman 1986: 11). The data become cases of larger categories by applying theoretical models to them; theory is the outcome of a theorization of your data, you 'theorise them into a case', so to speak. As Shulman (1986) points out: 'Generalisation does not inhere in the case, but in the conceptual apparatus of the explicator' (Shulman 1986: 12). This is an important point: generalization is perfectly possible, and it depends on the theoretical apparatus that you bring to bear onto your data including the theoretical frameworks studied prior to starting fieldwork that have been more or less determined by your particular research preparation and the formulation of your research goals. In my own work, both as a therapist and as a researcher, a psychosocial framework, involving understanding human beings as simultaneously biological, emotional, social and cultural, and positions the individual in networks of interpersonal relationships, organizations, and cultural/political/economic systems, has been crucial to practising intercultural art psychotherapy. It is an approach that encourages multi-disciplinarity and crosses the disciplinary boundaries that hinder the development of the knowledge and evidence base for psychosocial practice in the public sphere. In practice, in the field it translates into a way of working that is congruent with a collaborative participatory approach in humanitarian fieldwork (ALNAP, Groupe URD 2009) and the Mental Health and Psychosocial Support Programming for Refugee Operations guidelines issued by the UNHCR (2013). In relation to the experience of transgenerational migration, my generalizations will be about such issues and my case studies will belong to a larger category of psychosocial research. As Blommaert and Dong Jei (2010) observe, this does not occur just at the end of the research trajectory, as theoretical frameworks have been explored prior to starting your fieldwork, and many of the choices made in the process of formulating the research aims (what you hope to achieve) and objectives (the steps you take to achieve your aims).

Discussion

My ongoing research necessarily involves an examination of the approaches and processes outlined in this chapter. Exploratory workshops with art therapy students on the subject of transgenerational identity in relation to objects have proved illuminating in exploring processes of translation between media in art psychotherapy.

Understanding of the role of the intermediaries who perform the work of translation

1   In the case of art psychotherapy, this involves the triangular relationship between client/therapist in relationship to each other and to the image (Schaverien 1991) and the relationship of the image to the mental image (Bolle 2015).
2   In ethnography planned group discussions involving objects provide an accessible way to explore transgenerational cultural translation, encourage sharing and increase the potential to generate dialogue and discussion (O' Reilly 2005).

Reflection on the vehicles of translation, such as narratives, performances, objects and other cultural artefacts

1   In art psychotherapy, the image or object produced within or brought to the therapeutic setting, functions as a vehicle of translation as does its accompanying narrative and the potential therein for elaboration and exploration
2   In the object workshops these same processes were at play but in the very different context of planned discussions with already existing groups of people who knew each other and had some relation to the topic I was pursuing (O'Reilly 2009: 76). On no occasion was the proposition that experiences of transgenerational migration could be mediated through an engagement with objects or images, responded to as anything out of the ordinary (Williams 1989).

The transcription of discussion groups and interviews is ongoing and involves another layer of translation, from object to narrative, Spanish to English. However, preliminary findings suggest:

1   that making links between object, image and developing accompanying reflective narratives is not a rarefied pursuit but a very ordinary human phenomenon that can be successfully incorporated into participatory ethnographic research.

2   that most of these object narratives are about meaningful relationships with people, which concurs with Miller's finding '. . . that the people who successfully forge meaningful relationships to things are often the same as those who forge meaningful relationships with people, while those who fail usually also fail at the other, because the two are much more akin and entwined than is commonly appreciated'.

(Miller 2008: 105)

Notes

1   Translated from the original Spanish by the author.
2   Authors field notes.

Bibliography

ALNAP, Groupe URD (2009), *Participation Handbook for Humanitarian FieldWworkers – Involving Crisis-affected People in a Humanitarian Response*, Available online at: www.alnap.org/resource/8531 (accessed 19 July 2015).

Anderson, L. (2006), 'Analytic autoethnography', *Journal of Contemporary Ethnography*, 35 (4): 373–95.

Arber, A. (2006), 'Reflexivity: a challenge for the researcher as practitioner?', *Journal of Research in Nursing*, 11 (March): 147–57.

Atkinson, P. (2006) 'Rescuing autoethnography', *Journal of Contemporary Ethnography*, 35 (4): 400–4.

Austin, D. (2003), 'Community-based collaborative team ethnography: A community-university-agency partnership', *Human Organization*, 62 (2): 143–52.

Baily, Samuel L. (1999), *Immigrants in the Lands of Promise: Italians in Buenos Aires and New York City, 1870 to 1914*, Ithaca, NY: Cornell University Press.

Benjamin, W. (2006), *Berlin Around 1900*, London: Belknap.

Bergold, J. (2007), 'Participatory Strategies in Community Psychology Research—a Short Survey', in A. Bokszczanin, (ed.) *Poland Welcomes Community Psychology: Proceedings from the 6th European Conference on Community Psychology*, Opole: Opole University.

Bergold, J. & Thomas, S. (2012), 'Participatory Research Methods: A Methodological Approach in Motion', *Forum: Qualitative Social Research*, [S.l.], 13 (1). Available online at: www.qualitative-research.net/index.php/fqs/article/view/1801/3334> (accessed 21 August 2015).

Bird, J. (2012), 'Towards Babel: Language and Translation in Art Therapy', in H. Burt (ed.) *Art therapy and postmodernism: Creative Healing Through a Prism*, London: Jessica Kingsley.

Blommaert, J. & Dong Jie (2010), *Ethnographic Fieldwork, A Beginner's Guide*, Bristol: Multilingual Matters.

Bolle, R., Narducci, A., Palumbo, M., Poli, S. & Staroszynski, T (2007), *Intercultural Integraton and Art Therapy Handbook of Good Practice*, Florence: Tipografia DueP.

Bourdieu, P. (1990), *In Other Words: Essays Towards a Reflexive Sociology*, Stanford: Stanford University.

Bourdieu, P. & Wacquant, L. J. D. (1992), *An Invitation to Reflexive Sociology*, The University of Chicago.

Burdett, C. (2014), *Transnationalizing Modern Languages: Mobility, Identity and Translation in Modern Italian Cultures*. Available online at: www.transnationalmodernlanguages. ac.uk/about/project (accessed 22 August 2015).

Cacopardo, M.C. & Moreno, J. L. (1984), Caracteristicas demográficas y ocupacionales de los migrantes hacia Argentina (1880–1930), *Studi emigrazione*, 21 (75): 277–93.

Charmaz, K. (2006), 'The Power of Names', *Journal of Contemporary Ethnography*, 35 (4): 396–99.

Cheney, K. (2011), 'Children as ethnographers: reflections on the importance of participatory research in assessing orphans' needs', *Childhood*, 18 (2): 166–79.

Christian, P. J. (2012) *Gatekeepers in Conflict Research Settings: Ethics, Access & Safety*. Available online at: www.academia.edu/1494659/Gatekeepers_in_Conflict_ Research_Settings_Ethics_Access_and_Safety (accessed 7 June 2013).

Cook, T. (2012), 'Where participatory approaches meet pragmatism in funded (health) research: The challenge of finding meaningful spaces'. *Forum Qualitative Sozial-forschung/Forum: Qualitative Social Research*, 13 (1), Art. 18. Available online at: http// nbn-resolving.de/urn:nbn:de:0114-fqs1201187 (accessed 7 August 2015).

Denzin, N. (2006), 'Analytic Autoethnography, or Déjà Vu all Over Again', *Journal of Contemporary Ethnography*, 35 (4): 419–28.

Departamento de Derecho y Ciencias Políticas de la Universidad Nacional de La Matanza (2011), *Historias de inmigrantes italianos en Argentina*. Available online at: http://argentinainvestiga.edu.ar/noticia.php?titulo=historias_de_inmigrantes_italian os_en_argentina&id=1432#.VdscXrxVikp (accessed 24 August 2015).

Devoto, F. J. (1984) 'Las sociedades italianas de ayuda mutua en Buenos Aires y santa Fe: Ideas y Problemas', *Studi emigrazione*, 21 (75): 320–42.

Devoto, F. J. (2006), *Historias de los Italiano en Argentina*, Buenos Aires, Editorial Biblos.

Ellis, C. (2004), *The Ethnographic I: A Methodological Novel About Autoethnography*, Walnut Creek, CA: AltaMira.

Ellis, C., & Bochner. A. P. (2000), 'Autoethnography, personal narrative, reflexivity: Researcher as Subject', in Denzin N. K. & Lincoln, Y. S. (eds.) (2000), *Handbook of Qualitative Research*, (2nd edn.), Thousand Oaks, CA: Sage.

Epolito, G. (2011), 'Golondrinas: Birds of Passage – The Influence of Italianità in Art and Architecture of the Rio de La Plata Basin in the 19th and 20th Centuries', in Massari, S., Orsitto, F. & Spani, G. (eds.) (2001), *Italy, the Mediterranean . . . And Beyond*, Atti della conferenza Echioltremare, Roma 2011 (eds.), Isime-Casa Delle Letteratura.

Finlay, L. (2008), *Reflecting on 'Reflective practice'*, PBPL 52, The Open University.

Flyvbjerg, B (2006), 'Five misunderstandings about case-study research', *Qualitative Inquiry*, 12 (2): 219–45.

Forsdick, C. (2014), *Translating Cultures, Theme Overview.* Available online at: www.ahrc.ac.uk/Funding-Opportunities/Research-funding/Themes/Translating-Cultures/Pages/Translating-Cultures.aspx (accessed 18 September 2014).

Friedman (1994), *Cultural Identity and Global Process*, Sage.

Geertz, C. (1973), *The Interpretation of Cultures*, New York: Basic.

Hills de Zárate, M. (2010), Tropical Path (Part 1): The Life and Work of Antonia Eiriz, *ATOL: Art Therapy Online*, 1 (1) 2010 ATOL Available online at: http://journals.gold.ac.uk/119/3/Hill_Tropical.pdf (accessed 30 August 2015).

Hills de Zárate, M. (2011a), 'Tropical Path (Part 2): The Life and Work of Antonia Eiriz', *ATOL: Art Therapy Online*, 1 (2) 2011. Available online at: http//journals.gold.ac.uk/263/1/Tropical_Path2_Part_2.pdf (accessed 30 August 2015).

Hills de Zárate, M. (2011b) 'Arterapia: un Enfoque Psicosocial', in M. Marinovic & Reyes, P. (eds.), *Arteterapia – Reflexiones y Experiencias para un campo profesional*, Chile: TEHA.

Hocoy, D. (2002), 'Cross-cultural issues in art therapy', *Art Therapy: Journal of the American Art Therapy Association*, 19 (4): 141–5.

Hocoy, D. (2005), 'Ethnography as metaphor in psychotherapy training', *American Journal of Psychotherapy*, 59 (): 101–18.

Hocoy, D. (2006), 'Art therapy: working in the borderlands', *Art Therapy: Journal of the American Art Therapy Association*, 23 (3): 132–5

Hoey, B. A. (2014), *A Simple Introduction to the Practice of Ethnography and Guide to Ethnographic Fieldnotes*, Marshall University Digital Scholar (pp. 1–10).

Hogan, S. (2015) 'Lost in Translation: Intercultural Exchange in Art Therapy', in S. L. Brooke & C. E. Myers (eds.), *Therapists Creating a Cultural Tapestry: Using the Creative Therapies Across Cultures?*, Springfield: Charles C Thomas.

Hogan, S. & Pink, S. (2010), 'Routes to interiorities: art therapy and knowing in anthropology', *Visual Anthropology*, 23: 158–74, London: Routledge.

Israel, B. A., Eng, E., Schulz, A. J. & Parker, E. (eds.) (2013), *Community-Based Participatory Research for Health* (2nd edn), San Francisco: Jossey-Bass.

Jeffrey, B. & Troman,G. (2004), 'Time for ethnography', *British Educational Research Journal*, 30 (4): 535–48.

Lassiter, L. (2000), 'Authoritative texts, collaborative ethnography & native American Studies', *The American Indian Quarterly*, 24 (4): 601–14.

Lincoln, Y. S. & Guba, E. G. (1985), *Naturalistic Inquiry*, London: Sage.

Mignone, M. B. (2008), *Italy Today: Facing the Challenges of the New Millennium*, New York: Peter Lang.

Miller, D. (1983), 'Things Ain't What They Used to Be', *Royal Anthropological Newsletter* 59: 5–17.

Miller, D. (2005), *Materiality*, Durham, North Carolina: Duke University.

Miller, D. (2008), *The Comfort of Things*, Cambridge: Polity.

Miller, D. (2010), *Stuff*, Cambridge: Polity.

O'Reilly, K. (2009), *Key Concepts in Ethnography*, Sage.

Pace, S. (2012), 'Writing the Self into Research: Using Grounded Theory Analytic Strategies in Autoethnography', in N. McLoughlin & D. L. Brien (eds.) *TEXT Special Issue: Creativity: Cognitive, Social and Cultural Perspectives*. Available online at: www.textjournal.com.au/speciss/issue13/Pace.pdf (accessed 21 August 2015).

Parrado, E.A., McQuiston, C. & Flippen, C.A. (2005), 'Participatory survey research – Integrating community collaboration and quantitative methods for the study of gender and HIV risks among Hispanic migrants', *Sociological Methods and Research*, 34 (2): 204–39.

Parthasarathy, B. (2008), *The Ethnographic Case Study Approach*. Available online at: www.globalimpactstudy.org/2008/07/the-ethnographic-case-study-approach/ (accessed 22 August 2015).

Sanders, M. N. (2006), 'Gatekeeper', in V. Jupp (ed.) *The Sage Dictionary of Social Research methods*, London: Sage.

Scarzanella, E. (1981), 'L'industria argentina e gli immigrati italiani: nascita della borghesia bonarense', *Annali della Fondazione Luigi Einaudi*, 15: 365–412.

Schaverien, J. (1991), *The Revealing Image: Analytical Art Psychotherapy in Theory and Practice*, London and Philadelphia: Jessica Kingsley.

Schaverien, J. (2005), 'Inheritance: Jewish Identity, Art Psychotherapy Workshops and the Legacy of the Holocaust Mediated', in D. Dokter (ed.), *Arts Therapists, Refugees and Migrants*, London: Jessica Kingsley.

Schneider, A. (2000), *Futures Lost: Nostalgia and Identity among Italian Immigrants in Argentina*, Bern, Switzerland: Peter Lang.

Seeley, K. M. (1999), *Cultural Psychotherapy: Working with Culture in the Clinical Encounter*, New York: Jason Aronson.

Seeley, K. M. (2004), 'Short-term intercultural psychotherapy: ethnographic inquiry', *Social Work*, 49 (1): 121–30.

Shulman, L. S. (1986), 'Those who understand: knowledge growth in teaching', *Educational Researcher*, 15 (2): 4–14.

Shweder, R. A. (1991), *Thinking through cultures: Expeditions in cultural psychology*, Cambridge, MA: Harvard University.

Stedmon, J. & Dallos, R. (2009), *Reflective Practice in Psychotherapy and Counselling*, Open University.

Tedlock, B. (1991), 'From participant observation to the observation of participation: the emergence of narrative ethnography', *Journal of Anthropological Research*, 47, (1): 69–94.

Tsoi Hoshmand, L. (1996), 'Cultural psychology as meta-theory', *Journal of Theoretical and Philosophical Psychology*, 16 (1): 30–48.

Tsoi Hoshmand, L. (2005), 'Narratology, cultural psychology, and counseling research', *Journal of Counseling Psychology*, 52 (2): 178–86.

Tsoi Hoshmand, L. (2006), *Culture, Psychotherapy, and Counseling: Critical and Integrative Perspectives*, Thousand Oaks, California: Sage.

Turkle, S. (2011), *Evocative Objects: Things We Think With*, Cambridge, Massachusetts: MIT.

United Nations Refugee Agency (UNHCR) (2013), *Operational Guidance Mental Health and Psychosocial Support Programming for Refugee*, Geneva, Switzerland: The UN Refugee Agency.

Whitehead, (2005), 'Basic Classical Ethnographic Research Methods, Secondary Data Analysis, Fieldwork, Observation/Participant Observation, and Informal and Semi-structured Interviewing'. *Ethnographically Informed Community and Cultural Assessment Research Systems (EICCARS) Working Paper Series*. Available online at: www.cusag.umd.edu/programs/cehc/EICCARS (accessed 28 July 2015).

Williams, R. (1989), *Culture is Ordinary, in Resources of Hope: Culture, Democracy, Socialism*, London: Verso.

Woodward, S. (2013), 'Material Culture'. Available online at: www.oxford bibliographies.com/view/document/obo-9780199766567/obo-9780199766567–0085.xml (accessed 22 August 2015).

Chapter 10

Translating the cultural subtext

An auto-ethnographical narrative of facilitating a reflective space through creative methods for newly qualified teachers

Julianne Mullen-Williams

Introduction and context for research

In this chapter I present the trajectory of my experience as a researcher using auto-ethnography as a methodology to capture and contain some of the cultural aspects of the transferential processes that were revealed through my encounter with the newly qualified teacher participants. I will discuss how the methods of dramatherapy supervision, employed within the fieldwork sessions, offer an additional cultural frame of reference that highlights the transcendent influence of culture and transgenerational material on the potential motives of the researcher, notably Anglo-Irish relations. Transgenerational memory hypothesizes that some people unknowingly inherit the secret psychic substance of their ancestors 'lives' (McCoy-Wilson 2007). It will offer a brief literature review on other research that has incorporated auto-ethnography as a research method, and will share extracts from the findings of this particular method within this study.

For the purpose of clarity this chapter will be divided into vignettes in italics and commentary. The narrative vignettes are based on notes taken from reflections on the fieldwork sessions, insights drawn from discussions with my academic supervisor and creative artefacts devised and considered in the clinical supervision of the fieldwork, facilitated by a dramatherapy supervisor.

This research project uses auto-ethnography as a method to explore the impact of the researcher's cultural background on the research and its efficacy as a research tool. Within the therapeutic landscape, therapists, psychologists, counsellors, social workers and nurses, to name but a few, are obliged to engage in supervision with an external and more experienced practitioner to reflect on their practice as a gateway to understanding the world of their clients more clearly, so that they can provide the most appropriate support for them (Tselikas-Portmann 1999). There are many models of supervision in the helping professions that draw from different theoretical orientations: psychoanalysis, systems approach, creative and action methods. However, they all share a common purpose – to protect the best interests of the client (Hawkins & Shohet 2012) and thus improve professional competence through facilitating the supervisee(s) to reflect upon and learn from their practice. The encounter with the client can trigger some of the therapist's personal emotional, relational, cultural and psychological material. This phenomenon is referred to as counter-transference within psychodynamic orientations. One of the prominent functions of supervision is to delineate the therapist's counter-transference from the client's transference in order to provide the best support and care for the client. Dramatherapy supervisors Jones & Dokter (2008) cite the significance of the interaction between the therapeutic relationship and the personal histories of the therapist, client and supervisor as all being interrelated.

The British Association of Dramatherapy aims for supervision to develop and guarantee self-efficacy, as well as cultivating a reflective practitioner (Jones & Dokter 2008). Dramatherapy supervision is informed and underpinned by theories from the worlds of theatre, anthropology and psychology (Tselikas-Portmann 1999; Chesner & Zografou 2014; Jones & Dokter 2008).

Dramatherapy supervision utilizes creative methods to gain insight and a deeper understanding of the situation. The word metaphor in Greek means to 'carry across', indicating a transfer of meaning from one frame of reference to another. Grainger upholds that metaphor interprets whatever we want to talk about, that it escapes our logical grasp into its own unique way of transmitting these things, which are none the less real and true for being impossible to pin down: 'it was as if', 'it felt as though', or simply 'I can't describe what it was like – it was mind-blowing' (Grainger 2004:6). Creativity and the use of metaphor enable the supervisee to gain an aerial view of the situation they are exploring through which to observe the parallel process in the therapist's counter-transference. At times the dynamics of the relationship between the therapist and the client may be mirrored in the supervisory relationship in what has been referred to as a 'parallel process' (Eckstein & Wallenstein 1958; Hawkins & Shohet 2012; Faugier 1992). Jung (1965) believed that metaphor was one way of rendering the unconscious conscious for the growth of both himself and his clients.

When applied to the supervisor–supervisee relationship, creative methods can illuminate the struggles occurring in the therapeutic relationship between the therapist and the client. This maintains the safety of the client and develops the supervisee's sense of self-efficacy. Jenkyns (1997) advocates that the therapist rigorously monitor and analyse their own process, as it contains the nucleus of the work with the client. This nucleus holds information that is mirrored in other relationships: the client and their family, the therapist and the client, the therapist and the supervisor, the therapist/supervisor and their personal relationships.

Supervision can have a positive impact on dramatherapists (Jones and Dokter 2007), psychotherapists (Wheeler and Richards 2007) and social workers

(Bogo & McKnight 2006), although there is a dearth of evidence-based research to support findings. Sommer *et al.*'s (2010) qualitative study on the use of story in supervision demonstrates that metaphoric supervision appears to offer possibilities for assisting supervisees with self-reflection; however, there is still much to be learned about this process. Cashwell and Dooley's (2001) study on self-efficacy in supervision indicated the sustaining nature of supervision for practitioners: those receiving supervision were seeking professional licence, whereas the group not receiving supervision were not. This could be indicative of supervision supporting retention rates among therapists. Within dramatherapy supervision, wherein supervision is a compulsory component of state registration, 100 per cent of the respondents agreed supervision was integral to their practice and their careers (Jones and Dokter 2008).

The importance of self-efficacy and reflective practice is acknowledged in the teaching profession (Johnson & Birkeland 2003; Skaalvik & Skaalvik 2010). Riley (2011: 1) promotes the importance of relationships: relationship from the student's standpoint, relationship from the teacher's standpoint and *the priority given to relationship formation and maintenance from school leadership* that buttress the academic outcomes of grades. Recent English educational reforms have impacted on the research. Rising concerns about teacher retention rates are reaching crisis point in the UK (Hodgson 2014; DfE Research Report 151, September 2011: 81). The Association for Teachers and Lecturers' qualified members' survey states that over three-quarters of trainee teachers and newly qualified teachers have already considered leaving the profession due to an excessive workload (ATL January 2015). Deteriorating student discipline, lack of time for discussion and reflection, large class sizes, too many national initiatives and an overloaded, unmanageable curriculum have been cited as some of the contributing factors to a teacher shortage in England (MacBeath 2011).

These findings resonated with my own experience as an Irish teacher working in the UK, and have been the springboard for my doctorate research to ascertain if methods from the supervision of dramatherapy can translate to an educational context and augment the occupational psychology of newly qualified secondary school teachers. Occupational psychology pertains to the stress-inducing variables of the teaching profession: how workload, emotional labour and educational reform impact on job satisfaction and efficacy (Van Horn 2004). Emotional labour refers to having to behave in a professional and caring manner at all times, regardless of how one actually feels (Riley 2011: 43). Although it is an integral reality of teaching and is rooted in the 'caring' nature of being a teacher, if unrecognized it can have implications for teachers remaining in the profession (Isenbarger & Zembylas 2006).

Research design

The research took place in a Catholic secondary school with two consecutive groups of ten NQTs, who received dramatherapy informed 'supervision' during the first year of teaching alongside the standard school mentoring between 2012 and 2014. This chapter focuses on Group 1, from Nov 2012 to July 2013. It entailed facilitating one-hour fortnightly supervision sessions as part of the NQT induction programme. Participants were invited to take part in the research, and informed consent was procured. NQTs were given the option to withdraw at any stage throughout the process. The overall study is a mixed-method inquiry. Qualitative methodology included fieldwork notes of group supervision sessions and post-intervention individual semi-structured interviews, using interpretative phenomenological analysis. The quantitative measurements used to triangulate findings include the Teacher Sense of Efficacy Scale (Tschannen-Moran & Woolfolk Hoy 2007), The Brief Cope (Carver 1997) and the Teaching Satisfaction Scale (Ho & Au 2006), which were administered pre-, mid- and post-intervention. Auto-ethnography is one of the qualitative research methods used to analyse the impact of the researcher's process on the findings to aid verification of data.

Data collection methods for this auto-ethnography included notes on personal reflections after each session, from clinical supervision training, clinical supervision of the fieldwork, academic supervision and a diary of artefacts from personal therapy that included play-text extracts, stories and reading material from previous learning. Field notes help researchers become aware of the limiting nature of memory and bring details to the 'schematic landscape outline', which 'help fill in the richness, nuance, and complexity of the landscape, returning the reflecting researcher to a richer, more complex, and puzzling landscape than memory alone is likely to construct' (Chang 2008: 6).

Methods of data analysis for auto-ethnography method include cycles of analyses and interpretation of all data that pertain to insights regarding the cultural background of the researcher through interaction with the participants. Chang (2008: 9) refers to auto-ethnographic data analysis and interpretation as involving 'moving back and forth between self and others, zooming in and out of the personal and social realm, and submerging in and emerging out of data'. This pendulum of reflexivity continued during and after the fieldwork.

The writing style of this auto-ethnography includes what Van Maanen (1988) classifies as 'realist, confessional and impressionist tales', and Chang (2008) refers to as the focus of the realist being on facts and descriptions of those being observed. The 'confessional' includes the researcher's own personal biases and character flaws. My reflections are based on this narrative style, interwoven with thoughts, reflections and extracts from play-texts that resonate with the findings. Some of the auto-ethnographic analyses took part unconsciously while writing this chapter, revealing a 'storytelling style' that unconsciously mirrored a cultural 'Irish storytelling' trait (Hogan 1998). 'In using oneself as an ethnographic exemplar, the researcher is freed from the traditional conventions of writing. One's unique voicings – complete with colloquialisms, reverberations from multiple relationships, and emotional expressiveness – is honored' (Gergen & Gergen 2002: 14). The structure of the ethnographic notes is a dialogue between my own personal reflections on the sessions with the NQTs, the experiences of the NQTs and discoveries from a deeper examination of the work within my own supervision. The foray of insights and ruminations is punctuated by analyses and interpretations.

Rationale for auto-ethnography

Ethnographic approaches are immediately relevant to the dynamic and relational nature of dramatherapy supervision (Henning-Stout 1999). Stewart advocates ethnographically informed methods in psychology. She notes that ethnographic methods are 'compatible' with the 'methodological values' of most psychologists (2003: 3). Her work supports the idea that ethnographically informed methods enable researchers to place the experiences of individuals within a social context and have a hermeneutic design (Schon 1983), a conversation with the situation. Suzuki et al. (2005) commend auto-ethnography as a method for obtaining specific cultural data on belief and value systems in psychotherapy.

Where such philosophers as Husserl (Jones 1975; Klein & Westcott 1994; Osborne 1994; Polkinghorne 1983) promote 'bracketing out' prejudices prior to inquiry, Heidegger (1962) highlights the impossibility of this. Heidegger believes that we act within a background of bodily, personal and cultural practices that are always present (Laverty 2003). Acknowledging the concept of being 'in-between' can both cause uneasiness and transmute the experience of all who engage in the process and enhance the quality of the research (Siddique 2011). Such prejudices, formed in tradition, are integral to our being and enable and limit our understanding as we engage with our own biases (Denzin & Lincoln 2000; Diekelmann 2005; Koch 1996). Confronting our biases can be self-transformative and healing (Esping 2011; Wright 2009; Chang 2008; Smith 2005).

The drawbacks of using this method include becoming over-focused on the self-narrative at the expense of the culture that is being researched, the very cornerstone of ethnographic inquiry. Chang (2008) reminds auto-ethnographers to support their data and not rely solely on their own personal narrative. She argues that auto-ethnography should be ethnographical in its methodological orientation, cultural in its interpretive orientation, and autobiographical in its content orientation. Its primary goal is the procurement of an ethical cultural understanding through underlying autobiographical experience. Clandinin and Connelly (2000) challenge auto-ethnographers on their adherence to confidentiality. They question the ownership and subsequently the confidentiality of researchers' stories when it involves others. Denzin and Lincoln (2000) state that ethnographers have been criticized for generalizing findings to entire societies, on the basis of the study of only a few community members.

Auto-ethnography research

Within the health-psychology field auto-ethnography was used to investigate the phenomena of eating behaviour and eating disorders (Smith 2004). Within community psychology, Langhout (2006) used auto-ethnography to reflexively review her research and consider issues of race, class and gender. Woodward (2015) exercises auto-ethnography as a primary-research method into her experience of working as a Music Therapist in Bosnia and Herzegovina in post-repatriation.

Rozelle and Wilson (2012), in their ethnographic study on science-teacher trainees, advocate ethnography as a viable research method because it highlights what is happening on a microcosmic level, thus illuminating information about the world. However, Reed-Danahay (1997: 3) suggests that 'one of the main characteristics of an auto ethnographic perspective is that the auto ethnographer is a boundary-crosser and the role can be characterised as that of a dual identity'. My insights reflect the ebb and flow pattern of transition that occurs when moving from one stage of development to another: from student to teacher to researcher, from researcher to teacher to student. It has been my experience that, once we embark on a new stage, there is a purging of past experiences in order to make sense of the new terrain, as well as gaining more objectivity on the old and familiar. What unfolds between these shifting states from old to new is what Mitchell (1998) refers to as a 'liminal ritual', where unfinished business must be addressed.

Auto-ethnography findings

My autobiographical experience was multifarious, framed by a complex system of cultural and professional roles, norms and values. These were being deconstructed and re-framed through the interactions with the participants and the setting. I shared a parallel learning process with the teachers. I too was within an induction period, of becoming a supervisor,[1] which includes both an educative and learning function. Additionally, I was developing the necessary skills to be a researcher. Within the cohort of NQTs there were two first generation Southern Irish teachers. Distinguishing features of our shared parallels were a Catholic upbringing and post-colonial migration to the land of the former occupier.[2]

Moving in and out of these two roles of learner/supervisor and teacher/supervisor simultaneously accentuated recurring patterns of behaviour. These uncovered underlying motives for becoming a teacher and some of the hidden Anglo-Irish influences that buoyed these driving forces. Findings include personal notes and reflections (in italics) on the work with the NQTs from the early stages of the field research, followed by analysis and interpretations, which remain an open dialogue in supervision and personal therapy.

September 2011 – initial motives for becoming a teacher

Personal process notes

> *Kate*: I know those people from the back hills! I've taught them! Savages–
> that's what they are! And what pagan practices they have are no concern
> of ours – none whatever. It's a sorry day to hear talk like that in a Christian
> home, a Catholic home.
>
> (Dancing at Lughnasa by Brian Friel 1999: 29)

This quote reminds me of the power my Irish education wielded. School
was a safe and containing landscape abundant with opportunities for
creative expression, academic success, sporting achievement. Most
importantly it championed the development of individual potential, in
particular for women. It was peopled with Christians, experts and scholars
but above all it was a community pillared by firm but fair rules. A small
minority dared to challenge them but were subsequently defeated. When
I came upon the opportunity to train as a teacher in a foreign land I accepted
it, as I thought I would be returning to that nourishing isle of tutelage that
had served me so well. However, that script no longer existed. It had been
translated into a different tongue, populated with voices 'from the back
hills'. My unconscious sub-textual objective was to steadfastly re-create the
former text and assign the very same roles to the present cast of staff and
students. Inevitably the mission failed again and again. A call to adventure
steered me to unpack the subtext[3] of my own educational experience which
entailed climbing those back hills and encountering those savages that
roamed that Dionysian landscape.

(Mullen 2012)

Interpretation and analyses of process

In the quote from Dancing at Lughnasa Kate, a school teacher in rural Ireland
in 1936, refers to the back hills and savages. This can be translated as the subtext
for an attempt to control her own restrained and repressed anger, in response
to the imposing industrial revolution that rendered her unemployed, as well as
a wider Catholic quest for a moral monopoly. The 'moral monopoly' refers to
the nascent power of the Catholic Church over the morals of the Irish nation
through control of the Irish mother. They exerted a moral discipline over
passions and instincts that centred on physical intimacy, hence the prohibition
of contraceptives until the 1980s and a lack of sex education until the 1960s
(Inglis 1998). The Catholic Church's quest may have been an attempt, like
Kate's, to eradicate the English cartoonist view of the Irish as 'the untamed
savages of the West' (Inglis 1998: 2).[4]

These austere notions lay dormant within my psyche for some time, although
they were unconsciously steering my professional career towards education and

becoming a teacher. It was only through beginning PhD research that my own subtext and motives for becoming a teacher began to surface. My initial aim was to investigate the underlying reasons behind the increasing attrition and decreasing retention rates within the teaching profession in the UK.

During my sixth year of teaching (while teaching at one of the new Academies)[5] my realizations about the shifting landscape of teaching were exhumed within my clinical supervision for my practice as a dramatherapist. The more dramatherapy work I did, the more I realized I needed support in my teaching role. My inner savages were beginning to emerge. The auto-ethnographic research process of reflexivity had begun and was testing my ability to be vulnerable (Custer 2014). This prompted further research into the phenomenon of 'teacher vulnerability', which is defined as feeling powerless, threatened and questioned by others without being able to properly defend oneself and not feeling in control of the tasks and processes they are responsible for as teachers (Kelchtermans 2005). This notion of vulnerability can be exacerbated by educational policy and reforms that are not congruent with the teachers' deeply held beliefs about 'good teaching' (Kelchtermans 2005, Nias 1999). A teacher's sense of identity or agency (i.e. their ability to have influence over their lives and environments) can be greatly affected.

I learned how this fractured identity can lead to an inability to create trusting learning environments against the political backdrop of a growing 'managerial profession with increased accountability' (Lasky 2005). It can give rise to vulnerability, which induces feelings of fear, powerlessness and defencelessness, which can lead in turn to burnout (Brouwers et al. 2011; Demerouti et al. 2001). This vulnerability can be referred to as cognitive dissonance (Festinger 1957; Aronson & Mills 1959; Rideout & Windle 2010) or contextual disso-nance[6] (Rosenberg 1977).

I was becoming aware of my own cognitive dissonance, especially within my professional relationships with male authority figures and my persistent drive to re-write the script of teaching and learning. 'This was not like the schools in Ireland,' Serendipitously, while walking past my line manager's office, I came across a book entitled 'Attachment Theory and the Teacher–Student Relation-ship' by P. Riley (2011). This voiced everything I was experiencing, but more interestingly it focused on the formation of the attachment style of the teacher and how that translated to the attachment dynamics in the classroom and the school.

This inspired me to embark on PhD research that would hopefully explain the growing attrition rates and could idealistically increase retention rates. The mission had begun – to rescue the English education system. It was not possible at this stage to identify the deeply ingrained cultural influences that surreptitiously navigated my motivation. It was through the facilitation of a reflective space for others that my own motives, vulnerabilities and cultural awareness or lack thereof were reflected back through the methodological lens of auto-ethnography.

Encountering the savages: teaching in disguise

January 2012 – personal reflections on supervision diploma course

'How heavy is this glass of water? The absolute weight doesn't matter. It depends on how long you try to hold it' (Hawkins & Shohet 2012: 30).

The notion of 'holding' as a significant aspect of supervision has become an enlightening learning curve for me during these skills sessions on the supervision training course when I felt empowered to place the glass down so both myself and the other supervisor trainee could look at it collaboratively. I also felt comfortable to take the risk of putting down the glass and allowing the supervisor in to share the experience of its contents.

This is in contrast to my previous experience of the supervisory relationship where I cast the supervisor in the role of the 'all knowing authority' on my clinical practice. This fear of not meeting my projected high standards has led me to censoring some of the material that I bring to the sessions. I then may end up becoming overwhelmed and saturated with client material. Notably, holding on to past material and an unwillingness to share the burden has been a prominent theme within my own personal narrative. It has been quite surprising to discover its manifestation within this supervision course.

November 2012 – personal reflections on session with NQTs

NQT session

I had very emotional discussions with S and P. S was upset about how different the schools are in London compared to Ireland. She was worried about confidentiality and how she may be judged by the other newly qualified teachers in the group.

P talks about feeling either really angry or really terrified. I had a very emotional interview with this particular teacher. She was very upset, crying but almost fuelled by rage at having to come to this group. I said it was her decision and explained that it was up to her whether or not she partakes in the research. I turned the dictaphone off half- way through the interview as I felt guilty that I was researching when someone was so clearly upset. I found it very difficult to do my notes after this session as I felt like I had encountered post-traumatic stress.

Interpretation and analyses of process

I wondered where the fear of authority and showing vulnerability, for both myself and the NQTs, had come from? What was the block to 'getting it wrong?' The NQTs and I shared a fear of allowing others to help with this burden. Youell (2006), from a psychodynamic stance, refers to the fear of the unknown as a defence against anxiety. Any query about my work or ability was so emotionally overwhelming that it was best avoided. It was only when I encountered the tears of two of the newly qualified teachers, one of whom shares the same cultural identity, that I became conscious of my avoidance. At the time I wanted to cross the boundary of supervisor into one of Irish teacher in London and say 'Yes I know, in Ireland it is different. There is respect for authority.'

Supervision reflections after NQT session

The themes that came up regarding the NQT distress and my counter-transference were linked to post-traumatic stress, illustrated by my inability to write the notes straight after the initial session. This prompted an exploration of the overwhelming feelings I experienced through the use of objects. I chose lots of toy soldiers and animals and sculpted them into a large heap, one on top of the other, to represent my experience of the NQT session. It was very much like the aftermath of a war or battle.

Something similar to the Apocalypse. All the wounded animals are lying in a mess. Where do you go first? Are there any survivors? How can we look at this as part of research when so many have been casualties of war. It took the session to dissect the pieces and see what was underneath. There was land, a stable foundation. There is no way the war can be undone or time reversed. A contained space needs to be created in which to observe, explore and really see what lies beneath the mess. The soldiers represent the teachers who are each given the task of each looking after a designated part of the rubble. There is space between the shared pieces. They have space to walk around. I am the guide or facilitator to this process. What have the soldiers experienced? How are they been looked after? They need encouragement, containment and courage to look at what is really there and know that this research is being held.

Personal reflections on process

This notion of the 'wounded soldier' resonated with me. I can recall feeling completely overwhelmed by emotions while teaching at the Academy previously mentioned. It was something that emerged many times in my clinical supervision. It also brought back my own experience of attending primary school, whereby I suffered from separation anxiety quite acutely during the first three years.

Only in recent weeks I have remembered my initial two years at school in Junior School whereby I pined each morning as I disembarked from my parents' car and made my way into my classroom. I recall being unable to articulate the reasons for my tears and fretting. I just didn't want to go into the unknown.

It was separation anxiety. My biggest fear was getting it wrong in class and angering my kindergarten teacher. She was very nice but was easily irritated if you got something wrong which she had explained several times. I recall the immense pressure of painstakingly endeavouring to write the number 2. It was a spectacle for the whole class, they were all willing me to get it right. Eventually I did. This anxiety extended to the domestic space wherein if I shared this difficulty at home it resulted in the questioning of the quality of the school – best to avoid. Nobody could bear to get it wrong. Perhaps this explains why I was obsessed with playing 'school' in the role of the teacher by myself, might I add. Through play I was in complete control in the role of the teacher and I was able to make sense of the day's events by replaying them. Little did I know I was manifesting a career into existence!

Personal reflections on NQT session

Themes in the session included coping with student behaviour that was defined as 'craziness' and included 'lots of fights in lessons'.

> The teachers feel that they are being treated as emotional punch bags. They are struggling to make sense of the students' behaviour. Student attitudes are clashing with the teachers' belief systems about education, they compare the school and the students to their own education. One Irish teacher commented on how when she was a student it was shameful to be sent out of the classroom for bad behaviour. Shame managed behaviour. They were invited to create an image that depicted the students of concern through a metaphor or story. One group chose to explore a difficult yr 8 class. They created a bouncy castle where the floor was constantly uneasy. They placed themselves among the teaching group. The students of concern were dominating the bouncing castle. The teachers' representations of themselves were smaller than the students. They entitled this image 'how to gain control?' This was followed by labelling the students with 'I need . . .' sentences. Very young needs such as 'I need a male figure,' 'I need attention.' The second group created an image of 4 horses in each corner of the paper to represent a challenging yr 9 group. "Apocalypse when?" was the title. They found it difficult to place themselves in the image. They received comments from the other nqts that included uncertainty as to who were the students and who were the staff. This led to insights from the second group who noted how maybe the horses represented the staff from the 'student' point of view and the apocalypse reference is the teachers' lack of optimism and their feelings of dread surrounding the students. The students in the images seem to be very infant like, they remind me of the NQTs. I wonder if the yr 8 and 9 students are feeling out of control and looking for boundaries and containment. P still felt frustrated that there was no perceived solution to the yr 8 group.

Awareness was not helpful. 'They are un-teachable and that they can't achieve' This prompted me to discuss the notion of being' good enough' for this group I often feel quite emotional with teacher P and that I have been a 'bad mother 'to her and that I can't help her. What does she need?

Interpretation and analyses of process

My initial stage of being a supervisor, alongside the teachers' early teaching experience, mirrored the Year 8 students' feelings of confusion and need for containment. The nebulous landscape of being newly qualified engendered an awakening of dormant unresolved business from previous learning experiences that needed addressing (Mitchell 1998). Within the developmental approach to supervision, the first stage is characterized by vulnerability and insecurity about the supervisee's ability to execute their new role (Stolenberg & Delworth 1987). This is emulated in Fuller and Brown's prolifically referenced teacher developmental model, which moves outwards from concerns about the self to concerns about others (Fuller & Brown 1975; Conway & Clarke 2003).

Throughout the process of discovering my own discord and disharmony I began to reflect on the wider historical, social and political contexts of its manifestation. Was I experiencing a transgenerational memory of deeply entrenched shame within the Irish psyche over the loss of control over the Irish language and education system during English occupation and the subsequent struggle to learn the imposed new language? Living and working in the UK for over ten years enabled me to begin to explore the history of the relationship between these two countries from a distance. I recall being very wary of not being 'good enough', when I first arrived in London to attend drama school. Much to my surprise I was commended for my skills and welcomed. It took a while to process that my experience did not reflect the past relationship of these two countries. I was potentially picking up on what Mac an Ghaill (2000) refers to as the inferior position for the Irish in Britain as 'colonial others', within the context of a shared life 'between migrants and the host' society at the imperial centre. This underlying inferiority complex unconsciously permeated my motivation for writing about the research in comparison to the free-flowing auto-ethnographic extracts, which wrote themselves (Gergen & Gergen 2002). The research writing was tainted by feelings of inadequacy and ineptitude.

Further reflection prompted me to question if this sense of inadequacy was provoked by feelings of guilt and shame that prowl the Irish psyche, for seeking further development and education outside the tribal domain.

In her book *The Ancestor Syndrome* (1998), French psychotherapist Schutzenberger has catalogued, through her use of the genosociogram, many examples of the repetition of trauma across generations. Biologist Rupert Sheldrake discusses the notion of 'morphogenetic resonance', the tendency for events to happen repeatedly in the same location. He maintains that the individual is deeply embedded in the wider 'energy' field and every aspect of the field is contained in the client (St. Just 2008). I considered the morpho-genetic resonance of the Irish psyche and its transgenerational attachment to the authoritarian roles of England and the Catholic Church.

Conclusions and recommendations for practice and further research

I did not realize how ingrained my cultural upbringing had been until I attained geographical distance, which mirrors the distancing effect used by theatre practitioners such as Brecht and dramatherapists who use drama with the sole purpose of de-familiarizing the familiar to encourage audience/clients to 'meet each new situation with a freshness that questions old knowledge'(Seymour 2010). Within the teaching profession, Jaworski (2006: 194) introduces the notion of the distancing effect to the idea of being critical in relation to practice. The distancing effect is the ability of the researcher 'to distance himself from practice to reflect on his practice in ways which took him deeper into the beliefs and personal theories influencing his practice'. My quest was to cultivate a similar educational experience to match the one I had during my education in Ireland. Philip Riley (2011) refers to the beliefs and theories influencing prac-tice as the attachment patterns among teachers, which motivate or draw them back to school even if not their own, in order to attempt to re-create the school they experienced or create the ideal school that they would like to have gone through.

Reflective practice with trainee and newly qualified teachers may help clarify their motivations to teach by focusing on perceived teaching ability and social utility and subsequently aid teacher retention rates (Fokkens-Bruinsma, M. & Esther T. Canrinus 2012). In my personal narrative, education fulfilled a parental role. However, as it was a surrogate figure and not the actual parent, it could never fill the void that I was unconsciously filling by accruing numerous qualifications. These insights have amplified my understanding of the NQT's experience and they have helped me end an unhealthy repetitive cycle in my own teaching career. Self-reflection and self-examination are the means to self-understanding and self-transformation (Florio-Ruane 2001; Nieto 2003).

Looking through the cultural lens provides a frame of reference for under-standing cultural dissonance[7] that occurs, as well as cognitive dissonance. Chang (2008) encourages researchers to appreciate that what makes auto-ethnography ethnographical is its ethnographic intent of obtaining a cultural understand-ing of self that is personally allied to others in the society. Most of the teachers in the study had had a cultural experience of education that differed from their own educational setting. It included religion, country of origin, type of education and the setting of teacher-practice experience. They were subse-quently teaching adolescents from a diverse range of cultural backgrounds. Auto-ethnography has heightened my awareness of the implications that cultural difference have on both students, teachers and pedagogy.

One of the challenges of using auto-ethnography was being mindful of all the NQTs' experiences and not solely the ones that shared my ethnic background. Despite the constant expedition of 'moving back and forth between self and others' (Chang 2008: 9), feeling nebulous and emotionally exhausting at times, using auto-ethnography as a method of research has provided some insight into my motivations as a researcher and unconscious bias while working in the field with newly qualified secondary school teachers. This method has helped me monitor the impact of my own 'social location' within the research and provided me with a wider lens, through which to better understand the teachers. It has enabled me to observe (my own motivations and 'prejudices'), the horizon influencing 'the range of vision that includes everything that can be seen from a particular vantage point' (Gadamer 1994: 302). The horizon is 'not a rigid boundary but something that moves . . . and invites one to advance further' (Gadamer 1994: 245). In this way, our horizons are dynamic and temporal, moving with our experiences in the world.

By bracketing my own subjective trajectory through this research method, I have been able to obtain a more objective perspective on the rest of the research and have endeavoured to detach my personal responses from the data. The use of auto-ethnography operated as a container for much of the interpersonal dynamics during the rest of the research, notably providing more clarity to ascertain the IPA analyses of the interview data. Through the use of auto-ethnography I have gained an 'insider' stance, which deepened my understanding of my own teacher role which contributed to comprehending the NQTs experience.

> *Lieutenant Yolland*: Poteen-poteen-poteen. Even if I did speak Irish I'd always be an outsider here, wouldn't I? I may learn the password but the language of the tribe will always elude me, won't it? The private core will always be . . . hermetic, won't it?
>
> (Translations by Brian Friel 1996: 416)

Notes

1   In order to begin the field work I undertook a Diploma in Clinical Supervision.
2   Ireland was under British occupation until the Anglo-Irish Treaty in 1921. The Treaty preceded the Republic of Ireland Act 1948 whereby Ireland formally ceased to be a member of the Commonwealth. Northern Ireland remains a member of the Commonwealth.
3   I interpret subtext as content such as strong emotions, and motives that reside beneath the surface of dialogue or text, feelings and thoughts that are implicit rather than explicit or in psychodynamic terms; counter-transference.
4   The structure of the Catholic Church in Ireland expanded beyond the realm of religion. It infiltrated and influenced politics, economics, education, welfare and media. Inglis (1998) argues that the Catholic Church usurped control in response to Catholics enduring oppression and discrimination during the Penal Laws. The penal laws were passed after the Reformation. They penalized the practice of the

Roman Catholic religion in both Britain and Ireland. The 'untamed savages' refer to the stereotypical image of the Irish within English media during after occupation.

5   The coalition government initiatives gave birth to Academies. This refers to a publically funded independent school system bound by a funding agreement with the government. It has autonomy regarding flexibility in the curriculum and clearly established accountability measures. It entails devolving as much day-to-day decision-making as possible to the front line (The White Paper 2010).

6   Cognitive dissonance refers to the difficulty in coping with situations that conflict with inner beliefs. If consonance is not achieved maladaptive and irrational behaviour may arise. Attempts to reduce dissonance include acquiring new information, changing attitudes and reducing the importance of the cognitions (McLeod 2008).

7   A phenomenon that may present itself when individuals that participate in multiple cultures (most of us) are faced with situations where s/he perceives conflicts between a set of rules from one culture and the rules of another. This phenomenon may even appear in the *same* culture (across "sub-cultures") (Youell 1999).

Bibliography

Adams, M. (2014), *The Myth of the Untroubled Therapist*, London: Routledge.

Aronson, E. & Mills, J. (1959), 'The effect of severity of initiation on liking for a group', *The Journal of Abnormal and Social Psychology*, 59 (2): 177–81.

Association of Teachers and Lecturers (ATL) (2015) *Conference Report*, Liverpool.

Bogo, M. & McKnight, K. (2006), Clinical Supervision in Social Work: a Review of the Research Literature', *The Clinical Supervisor*, 24 (1–2): 49–67.

Brouwers, A., Tomic, W., & Boluijt, H. (2011), 'Job demands, job control, social support and self-efficacy beliefs as determinants of burnout among physical education teachers', *European Journal of Psychology*, 7: 17–39.

Carver, C. S. (1997), 'You want to measure coping but your protocol's too long: Consider the Brief COPE', *International Journal of Behavioral Medicine*, 4: 92–100.

Cashwell, T. H. & Dooley, K. (2001), 'The Impact of Supervision on Counselor Self-efficacy', *Clinical Supervisor* 20 (1): 39–47.

Chang, H. (2008), *Auto-ethnography as a Method*, Pan Alto, CA: Left Coast.

Chesner, A. & Zografou, L. (2014), *Creative Supervision across Modalities*, London: Jessica Kingsley.

Clandinin, D. J. & Connelly, F. M., (2000), *Narrative Inquiry: Experience and Story in Qualitative Research*, San Francisco, CA: Jossey-Bass.

Conway, P. F. & Clark, C. (2003), 'The Journey Inward and Outward: A Re-examination of Fuller's Concerns-based Model of Teacher Development', *Teaching and Teacher Education*, 19 (5): 465–82.

Custer, D. (2014), 'Autoethnography as a transformative research method', *The Qualitative Report*, 19 (37): 1–13.

Demerouti, E., Bakker, A., Nachreiner, F. & Schaufeli, W. (2001), 'The job demands–resources model of burnout', *Journal of Applied Psychology*, 86: 499–512.

Denzin, N. K., & Lincoln, Y. S. (2000), 'Introduction: The Discipline and Practice of Qualitative Research', in N. K. Denzin & Y. S. Lincoln (eds.), *Handbook of Qualitative Research* (2nd edn., pp. 1–29). Thousand Oaks, CA: Sage.

Department for Education (2011), *A Profile of Teachers in England from the 2010 School Workforce Census*, DfE Research Report 151, September 2011: 81.

Diekelmann, J. (2005), 'The Retrieval of Method: The Method of Retrieval', in P. Ironside (ed.), *Beyond Method: Philosophical Conversations in Healthcare Research and Scholarship*, Madison: University of Wisconsin.

Eckstem, R. & Wallenstein, R. S. (1958), *The Teaching and Learning of Psychotherapy*, New York: Basic.

Esping, A. (2011), 'Autoethnography as logotherapy: an existential analysis of meaningful social science inquiry', *Journal of Border Educational Research*, 9 (Fall): 59–67.

Faugier, J. (1992), 'The Supervisory Relationship', in T. Butterworth and J. Faugier (eds.) *Clinical Supervision and Mentorship in Nursing*, London: Chapman and Hall.

Festinger, L. (1957), *A Theory of Cognitive Dissonance*, Stanford, CA: Stanford University.

Florio-Ruane, S. (2001), *Teacher Education and the Cultural Imagination*, Mahwah, NJ: Lawrence Erlbaum.

Fokkens-Bruinsma, M. & Canrinus, E. T. (2012), 'Adaptive and maladaptive motives for becoming a teacher', *Journal of Education for Teaching: International research and pedagogy*, 38 (1): 3–19.

Friel, B. (1996), *Brian Friel Plays 1*, London: Faber & Faber.

Friel, B. (1999), *Brian Friel Plays 2*, London: Faber & Faber.

Fuller, F. F. & Brown, O. H. (1975), 'Becoming a Teacher', in K. Ryan (ed.), *Teacher Education* (74th Yearbook of the National Society of Education, pp. 25–52), Chicago: University of Chicago.

Gadamer, H. G. (1994), *Truth and method* (2nd edn.), New York: Seabury.

Gergen, M. & Gergen, K. (2002), 'Ethnographic Representation as Relationship', in A. Bochner & C. Ellis (eds.), *Ethnographically Speaking: Autoethnography, Literature, and Aesthetic* (pp. 11–33), Walnut Creek, CA: Altamira.

Grainger, R. (2004), 'Theatre and encounter', *Dramatherapy*, 26 (1): 4–9.

Hawkins P. & Shohet, R. (2012), *Supervision in the Helping Professions* (4th edn.) Buckingham: Open University.

Heidegger, M. (1962), *Being and Time*, New York: Harper. (Original work published 1927).

Henning-Stout, M. (1999), 'Learning consultation: an ethnographic analysis', *Journal of School Psychology*, 37: 73–98.

Ho, C. L. & Au, W. T. (2006), 'Teaching satisfaction scale: measuring job satisfaction of teachers', *Educational and Psychological Measurement*, 66: 172–85.

Hodgson, P. (2014), DBE School Teachers' Review Body, Twenty-Fourth Report-2014. Available online at: www.gov.uk/government/uploads/system/uploads/attachment_data/file/318574/STRB_24th_Report_Cm_8886_web_accessible.pdf (accessed 30 August 2015).

Hogan, F. (1998), 'Soulful storytelling with men: an invitation to intimacy, in *Feedback – The Magazine of the Family Therapy Association of Ireland*, 8 (1): 17–22.

Inglis, T. (1998), *Moral Monopoly: The Rise and Fall of the Catholic Church in Modern Ireland*, Dublin: University College Dublin.

Isenbarger, L. & Zembylas, M. (2006), 'The Emotional Labour of Caring in Teaching', *Teaching and Teacher Education* 22: 120–34.

Jaworski, B. (2006), 'Theory and practice in mathematics teaching development: critical inquiry as a mode of learning to teach', *Journal of Mathematics Teacher Education* 9: 187–211.

Jenkyns, M. (1997), *The Play's The Thing*, London: Routledge.

Johnson, S. M. & Birkeland, S. E. (2003), 'The schools that teachers chose', *Educational Leadership*, 60 (8): 20.

Jones, P. & Dokter, D. (eds.) (2008), *Supervision of Dramatherapy*, London: Routledge.

Jones, W. T. (1975), *The Twentieth Century to Wittgenstein and Sartre* (2nd revised edn.), San Francisco, CA: Harcourt Brace Jovanovich.

Jung, C.G. (1965), *Memories, Dreams and Reflections*, New York: Random House.

Kelchtermans G. (2005), 'Teachers' Emotions in Educational Reforms: Self-understanding, Vulnerable Commitment and Micropolitical Literacy', *Teaching and Teacher Education* 21: 995–1006.

Klein, P. & Westcott, M. (1994), 'The changing character of phenomenological psychology', *Canadian Psychology*, 35 (2): 133–57.

Koch, T. (1996), 'Implementation of a hermeneutic inquiry in nursing: Philosophy, rigour and representation', *Journal of Advanced Nursing*, 24, 174-84.

Langhout, R. D. (2006), 'Where am I? Locating myself and its implications for collaborative research', *American Journal of Community Psychology*, 37: 267–74.

Lasky, S. (2005), 'A sociocultural approach to understanding teacher identity, agency and professional vulnerability in a context of secondary school reform', *Teaching and Teacher Education*, 21 (8): 899–916.

Laverty, S. M. (2003), 'Hermeneutic phenomenology and phenomenology: a comparison of historical and methodological considerations', *International Journal of Qualitative Methods*, 2 (3) Article 3. Available online at: www.ualberta.ca/~iiqm/back issues/2_3final/html/laverty.html (accessed 30 August 2015).

Mac an Ghaill, M. (2000), 'The Irish in Britain: the invisibility of ethnicity and anti-Irish racism', *Journal of Ethnic and Migration Studies* 26 (1): 137–47.

MacBeath J. (2011), 'Education of teachers: the English experience', *Journal of Education for Teaching: International Research and Pedagogy*, 37 (4): 377–86.

McCoy-Wilson, S. (2007), 'In "Rememory": beloved and transgenerational ghosting in black female bodies', Graduate English Association New Voices Conference 2007, Paper 5.

McIlveen, P. (2007), 'The genuine scientist-practitioner in vocational psychology: an autoethnography', *Qualitative Research in Psychology*, 4 (4): 295–311.

McLeod, S. A. (2008), Cognitive Dissonance. Available online at: www.simply psychology.org/cognitive-dissonance.html (accessed 30 August 2015).

Mitchell, S. (1998), 'The Theatre of Self-expression', *Dramatherapy*, 20 (1): 3–11.

Mullen (2012), 'Translating relational subtext: a method to augment the professional training of teachers', Paper presented at The British Association of Dramatherapists Annual Conference.

Nias, J. (1999), 'Teachers' Moral Purposes: Stress, Vulnerability, and Strength', in R. Vandenberghe and M. Huberman (eds.), *Understanding and Preventing Teacher Burnout: A Sourcebook of International Research and Practice* (pp. 223–37), Cambridge: Cambridge University.

Nieto, S. (2003), *What Keeps Teachers Going?* New York: Teachers College.

Osborne, J. (1994), 'Some similarities and differences among phenomenological and other methods of psychological qualitative research', *Canadian Psychology*, 35 (2): 167–89.

Polkinghorne, D. (1983), *Methodology for the Human Sciences: Systems of Inquiry*, Albany: State University of New York.

Reed-Danahay, D. E. (1997), *Auto/Ethnography: Rewriting the Self and the Social*, Oxford: Berg.

Rideout, G. & Windle, S. (2010), 'Beginning teachers' pupil control ideologies: an empirical examination of the impact of beliefs about education, mentorship, induction, and principal leadership style', *Canadian Journal of Educational Administration and Policy*, 104 (May).

Riley, P. (2011), *Attachment Theory and the Student-Teacher Relationship*, New York: Routledge.

Rosenberg, M. (1977), 'Contextual dissonance effects: nature and causes', *Psychiatry*, 40: 205–17.

Rozelle, J. J. & Wilson, S. M. (2012), 'Opening the black box of field experiences: how cooperating teachers' beliefs and practices shape student teachers' beliefs and practices', *Teaching and Teacher Education*, 28 (8): 1196–205.

St. Just, A. (2008), *A Question of Balance*, Heidelberg: Carl-Auer Systeme Verlag.

Schon, D. (1983), *The Reflective Practitioner. How Professionals Think In Action*, New York: Basic.

Seymour, A. (2010), 'Brecht in Italy', *Dramatherapy*, 31 (1): 15–20.

Siddique, S. (2011), 'Being in-between: the relevance of ethnography and auto-ethnography for psychotherapy research', *Counselling and Psychotherapy Research*, 11 (4): 310–16.

Skaalvik, E. M. & Skaalvik, S. (2011), 'Teacher job satisfaction and motivation to leave the teaching profession: relations with school context, feeling of belonging, and emotional exhaustion', *Teaching and Teacher Education*, 27 (6): 1029–138.

Smith, C. (2005), 'Epistemological intimacy: a move to autoethnograph', *International Journal of Qualitative Methods*, 4 (2), Article 6.

Sommer, C. A., Ward, J. E. & Scofield, T. (2010), 'Metaphoric stories in supervision of internship: a qualitative study', *Journal of Counseling and Development*, 88 (4): 500–7.

Stewart, A. J. (2003), 'Gender, race, and generation in a Midwest high school: using ethnographically informed methods in psychology', *Psychology of Women Quarterly*, 27: 1–11.

Stolenberg, C. & Delworth, U. (1987), *Supervising Counselors and Therapists: A Developmental Approach*, San Francisco: Jossey-Bass Wiley.

Suzuki, L. A., Ahluwalia, M. K., Quizon, C. A. & Mattis, J. S. (2005), 'Ethnography in counseling psychology research: possibilities for application, *Journal of Counseling Psychology by the American Psychological Association*, 52 (2): 206–14.

Tschannen-Moran, M. & Woolfolk Hoy, A. (2007), 'The differential antecedents of self-efficacy beliefs of novice and experienced teachers', in *Teaching and Teacher Education*, 23: 944–56.

Tselikas-Portmann E. (ed.) (1999), *Supervision and Dramatherapy*, London: Jessica Kingsley.

Van Horn, J. E., Taris, T. W., Schaufeli, W. B. & Schreurs, P. C. (2004), 'The structure of occupational well-being: a study among Dutch teachers', *Journal of Occupational and Organizational Psychology*, 77: 365–75.

Van Maanen, J. (1988), *Tales of the Field: on Writing Ethnography*, Chicago, IL: University of Chicago.

Wheeler, S. & Richards, K. (2007), 'The impact of clinical supervision on counsellors and therapists, their practice and their clients: a systematic review of the literature', *Counselling and Psychotherapy Research*, 7 (1): 54–65.

Woodward, A. M. (2015), 'Tapestry of tears: an autoethnography of leadership, personal transformation, and music therapy in humanitarian aid in Bosnia Herzegovina', *Dissertations and Theses*, Paper 192.

Wright, J. K. (2009), 'Autoethnography and therapy writing on the move', *Qualitative Inquiry*, 15: 623–40.

Youell, B. (2006), *The Learning Relationship*, London: Karnac.

Yowell, C. (1999), 'Cultural Dissonance as a Risk Factor in the Development of Students', in E. Gordon (ed.) *Education and justice: A View from the Back of the Bus*, New York: Teachers College.

Index

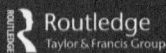